Basic Human Neuroanatomy

Basic Human Neuroanatomy

An Introductory Atlas

FOURTH EDITION

Craig Watson, M.D., Ph.D.

ASSOCIATE CLINICAL PROFESSOR
DEPARTMENTS OF NEUROLOGY AND HUMAN ANATOMY
UNIVERSITY OF CALIFORNIA, DAVIS,
SCHOOL OF MEDICINE

LITTLE, BROWN AND COMPANY
Boston　　　Toronto　　　London

To my students —
past, present, and future

Preface

This edition represents a major revision and expansion, but the objectives of the book remain unchanged. My goal is to provide a book that will meet the needs of a range of students that includes undergraduates, students in paramedical programs, medical students, graduate students, and residents studying for board examinations. The photographs in the Atlas (Part IV) are again labeled in a manner that allows and encourages self-study, self-testing, and review. I encourage students to refer regularly to the illustrations in Part IV when studying the text in Parts I, II, and III (and vice versa). Used in this way, the book can be helpful in the laboratory as well as at home for self-study and review.

I have revised Part II completely to present new information and current concepts concerning the major functional neuroanatomical pathways. In response to student suggestions, "pathway diagrams" have been included for each of the pathways described. The original diagrams have been redrawn and a total of 42 new illustrations have been added to this part of the book. The illustrations and angiograms in Part III have also been replaced and revised. In this section, nine illustrations have been added and six new angiograms replace those found in the Third Edition. In the Atlas portion of the book (Part IV) two photographs of the external anatomy of the brain stem have been included. Two coronal sections of the cerebrum have been added along with two new transverse sections of the brain stem stained with the Mulligan method. In the Weigert-stained transverse sections of the brain stem, two sections have been added. A coronal section of the hippocampal formation stained with the cresyl violet method is included in view of the increasing importance of this region of the brain in the understanding of learning and memory, Alzheimer's disease, and certain types of epilepsy. An accompanying illustration of the principal pathways and connections in the hippocampal formation has been included. Thirty new MRI scans have been placed opposite corresponding brain sections and include scans obtained in sagittal, horizontal, and coronal planes. I would encourage students to correlate structures seen in the brain sections with those clearly visible in this remarkable imaging modality that allows us to view exquisite brain anatomy in the living person. Illustrations have been placed opposite all the photographs of the Weigert-stained transverse sections of the spinal cord and brain stem. These illustrations define the position, extent, and relationships of many of the tracts and nuclei in the spinal cord and brain stem. Students may find it helpful to color-code the different pathways and nuclei in sequential spinal cord and brain stem sections to facilitate self-study and to develop a three-dimensional understanding of the pathways and structures in different regions of the brain and spinal cord. In view of recent developments in the field of chemical neuroanatomy, I have indicated the major sources of the principal neurotransmitter systems in the Atlas portion of the book. All in all, 71 illustrations, 11 photographs of the brain, and 30 MRI scans have been added to this edition.

Terminology throughout adheres to the *Nomina Anatomica* as adopted by the International Anatomical Nomenclature Committee in 1989. I urge all members of the medical community — students, teachers, and clinicians — to utilize this internationally adopted nomenclature to facilitate the transition to a uniform, logical, and informative terminology.

I am indebted to my colleagues, Vijaya K. Vijayan, M.B.B.S., Ph.D., and Ronan O'Rahilly, M.D., D.Sc., Department of Human Anatomy, University of California, Davis, School of Medicine, for their thoughtful suggestions and criticisms. Their input is greatly appreciated. In addition, Dr. O'Rahilly provided me with two brain stem sections originally belonging to our friend and colleague, the late Professor Ernest Gardner; and Dr. Vijayan obtained permission from James W. Geddes, Ph.D., Department of Psychobiology, University of California, Irvine, to use the coronal section of the hippocampal formation. I thank the many students who were kind enough to take the time and effort to review the Third Edition of this book and make suggestions for this edition. I also wish to thank Dr. Surl Nielsen, neuropathologist at Sutter Community Hospital and U.C. Davis, School of Medicine, for his help in the procurement and processing of the new brain sections, and Dr. William Keyes for his help in obtaining the new angiograms. The editorial assistance of Wayne Muller and Jaime Watson is also greatly appreciated. Special gratitude and admiration is extended to Craig Hillis for his painstaking creation of all of the illustrations in this edition and Gabriel Unda for his careful photographic work. Finally, I wish to thank Ms. Kristin L. Odmark of Little, Brown & Company for her enthusiasm, support, and assistance in this project.

C.W.
Sacramento, California

Contents

Part Three
BLOOD VESSELS OF THE BRAIN AND SPINAL CORD

Part Four
ATLAS OF THE BRAIN AND SPINAL CORD

Part One
Organization of the Nervous System

The Nervous System

The nervous system is an extremely complex organization of structures that serves as the main regulative and integrative system of the body. It receives stimuli from the individual's internal and external environments, interprets and integrates this information, and selects appropriate responses to it. The parts of the human nervous system that are highly developed (e.g., the cerebral cortex) allow us to use information in a much less stereotyped manner than can the other members of the animal kingdom, thereby presenting the opportunity for humane and cooperative behavior based on rational thought as well as the more automatic survival behavior characteristic of lower animals.

The nervous system can be divided arbitrarily, for the purpose of description, into two large divisions: the *central nervous system* and the *peripheral nervous system*. The central nervous system is composed of the brain and spinal cord, and the peripheral nervous system consists of the end organs, nerves, and ganglia that connect the central nervous system with all other parts of the body. The *autonomic (or involuntary) nervous system* is sometimes described as part of the peripheral nervous system, but it really is part of both the central and the peripheral nervous systems. However, to repeat, you should always remember that all these "divisions" are arbitrary and artificial and that the nervous system functions as an entity, not in parts. With that in mind, the organization of the nervous system can be summarized as follows:

Organization of the Nervous System

I. Central Nervous System (CNS)
  A. Brain
  B. Spinal cord
II. Peripheral Nervous System (PNS)
  A. Cranial nerves — 12 pairs
  B. Spinal nerves — 31 pairs
    1. Cervical — 8 pairs
    2. Thoracic — 12 pairs
    3. Lumbar — 5 pairs
    4. Sacral — 5 pairs
    5. Coccygeal — 1 pair
III. Autonomic Nervous System (ANS)
  Constituent part of CNS and PNS
  A. Parasympathetic (craniosacral) division
    1. Cranial part — related to cranial nerves III, VII, IX, X
    2. Sacral part — related to sacral cord levels and sacral spinal nerves 2, 3, 4
  B. Sympathetic (thoracolumbar) division
    1. Arises from the spinal cord from T_1 to L_2
    2. Forms the sympathetic trunk with its ganglia

THE CENTRAL NERVOUS SYSTEM

The brain and spinal cord are composed of many millions of nerve cells, or neurons, which are held together and supported by specialized nonconducting cells known collectively as *neuroglia*. Both parts of the central nervous system are composed of two types of tissue, *gray matter* and *white matter*. The gray matter is made up mainly of neuron cell bodies and their closely related processes (mainly dendrites), while the white matter consists of bundles of myelinated nerve fibers (mainly axons). Within the central nervous system, neurons make functional contact with one another by way of *synapses*, whereas they are functionally associated with the structures of the body by means of the peripheral nervous system. The various subdivisions of the embryonic central nervous system and their adult derivatives are shown below.

Divisions of the Central Nervous System

Embryonic Divisions	Adult Derivatives	Cavities
I. Brain		
A. Prosencephalon		
1. Telencephalon	Cerebral hemispheres	Two lateral ventricles
2. Diencephalon	Thalamus, hypothalamus	Third ventricle
B. Mesencephalon	Midbrain	Cerebral aqueduct
C. Rhombencephalon		
1. Metencephalon	Pons, cerebellum ⎱	
2. Myelencephalon	Medulla oblongata ⎰	Fourth ventricle
II. Spinal cord	Spinal cord	Central canal

THE PERIPHERAL NERVOUS SYSTEM

Nervous impulses are conveyed to and from the central nervous system by the various parts of the peripheral nervous system. *Afferent*, or *sensory*, *nerve fibers* carry impulses arising from the stimulation of sensory end organs (or receptors) toward the central nervous system; *efferent*, or *motor*, *fibers* carry impulses from the central nervous system to the effector organs (e.g., muscle fibers and glands). Some nerve fibers are associated with the structures of the body wall or the limbs, such as skeletal muscles, skin, bones, and joints. These fibers are called *somatic fibers* and are, of course, both afferent and efferent. Other fibers, also both afferent and efferent, are more closely associated with the internal organs, blood vessels, smooth muscle, and cardiac muscle. These fibers are referred to as *visceral fibers*. As a rule (but not always), most *peripheral nerves* contain all of the previously mentioned fibers (i.e., somatic efferent and somatic afferent, and visceral efferent and visceral afferent), and therefore it is rarely correct to speak of *sensory* or *motor nerves*. It is much more appropriate to use the term *muscular nerve* to describe a nerve supplying a muscle, since in addition to somatic motor fibers to the muscle, it contains somatic sensory fibers for muscle–tendon sensation (proprioception) as well as visceral afferent and visceral efferent fibers to the blood vessels of the muscle. In a like manner, a nerve supplying the skin should be called a *cutaneous nerve* because it contains visceral efferent and afferent fibers to blood vessels, arrector pili muscles, and sweat glands, as well as somatic sensory fibers for skin sensations. To confuse matters further, some of the structures in the head and neck (e.g., the eye, ear, nose, tongue, and the embryonic pharyngeal arch region) are classically referred to as *special* structures due to the fact that they are not present in the rest of the body. Because these structures are considered special, the structures found in the rest of the body (e.g., regular myotomic skeletal muscle, smooth muscle, glands, skin) are called *general*. So, we end up with *general* and *special, somatic* and *visceral, efferent* and *afferent* fibers in some peripheral nerves. Obviously, because the special fibers supply only head and neck structures, they are present only in (some) cranial nerves. General fibers, on the other hand, are present in both spinal and cranial nerves. All this gibberish falls under the general heading of the "functional components of peripheral nerves" and is summarized below for your reading pleasure.

Functional Components of Peripheral Nerves

A. Cranial and spinal nerves
  1. General somatic afferent (GSA) — Conscious sensation (e.g., pain, temperature, touch, proprioception)
  2. General visceral afferent (GVA) — Visceral sensation (mainly pain; also ischemia, blood pressure, etc.)
  3. General visceral efferent (GVE) — Autonomic motor to smooth and cardiac muscle and glands (parasympathetic and sympathetic; preganglionic and postganglionic)
  4. Somatic efferent (SE) — Voluntary motor to skeletal muscle (derived from myotomes)

B. Cranial nerves only
  5. Special visceral efferent (SVE) — Voluntary motor to skeletal muscle (derived from branchiomeres)
  6. Special visceral afferent (SVA) — Visceral sensations of taste and smell
  7. Special somatic afferent (SSA) — Somatic sensations of vision, hearing, and equilibrium

Functional Components of Cranial Nerves

Nerve	Functional Component	Structure Innervated	Location of Cell Bodies; First Synapse
Olfactory (I)	SVA — smell	Olfactory epithelium in nasal cavity	Nasal epithelium; olfactory bulb
Optic (II)	SSA — vision	Retina (rods and cones) of eye	Ganglion cells of retina; lateral geniculate body of thalamus
Oculomotor (III)	SE	Superior, medial, and inferior rectus, inferior oblique, and levator palpebrae superior Mm.	Oculomotor nucl.
	GVE — parasympathetic	Sphincter pupillae and ciliary Mm.	Accessory oculomotor nucl.; ciliary ganglion
Trochlear (IV)	SE	Superior oblique M.	Trochlear nucl.
Trigeminal (V)	GSA	Skin and mucosae of face and head via ophthalmic, maxillary, and mandibular divisions	Trigeminal ganglion; pontine nucl. and spinal nucl. of V
	SVE	Mm. of mastication, tensors tympani and veli palatini, mylohyoid, and anterior digastric Mm.	Motor nucl. of V
	GSA — proprioceptive	Same as for SVE	Mesencephalic nucl. of V
Abducent (VI)	SE	Lateral rectus M.	Abducent nucl.
Facial (VII)	SVE	Facial Mm., stapedius, stylohyoid, and posterior digastric Mm.	Facial nucl.
	GVE — parasympathetic	Lacrimal, sublingual, and submandibular glands; other minor glands and mucosal surfaces	Superior salivatory nucl.; pterygopalatine, submandibular, and diffuse submandibular ganglia
	SVA — taste	Taste buds of anterior two-thirds of tongue	Geniculate ganglion; nucl. of solitary tract
	GVA	Middle ear	Geniculate ganglion; nucl. of solitary tract
	GSA	External ear	Geniculate ganglion; spinal nucl. of V
Vestibulocochlear (VIII)	SSA — hearing	Spiral organ of cochlea	Cochlear (spiral) ganglion; cochlear nuclei
	SSA — equilibrium	Ampullae of semicircular ducts and maculae of saccule and utricle	Vestibular ganglion; vestibular nuclei
Glossopharyngeal (IX)	SVA — taste	Taste buds of posterior third of tongue	Inferior ganglion of IX; nucl. of solitary tract
	GVE — parasympathetic	Parotid gland	Inferior salivatory nucl.; otic ganglion
	GVA	Pharynx (gag reflex), carotid sinus, posterior third of tongue, auditory tube, and middle ear	Inferior ganglion of IX; nucl. of solitary tract
	SVE	Stylopharyngeus M.	Nucleus ambiguus
	GSA	External ear	Superior ganglion of IX; spinal nucl. of V

Nerve	Functional Component	Structure Innervated	Location of Cell Bodies; First Synapse
Vagus (X)	GVE — parasympathetic	Smooth and cardiac Mm. and glands of thoracic and abdominal organs through transverse colon	Dorsal nucl. of X; many terminal ganglia on, in, or near organs supplied
	GVA	Carotid and aortic bodies; all listed for GVE — parasympathetic	Inferior ganglion of X; nucl. of solitary tract
	SVE	Mm. of soft palate, pharynx, larynx, and esophagus	Nucleus ambiguus
	SVA — taste	Epiglottis	Inferior ganglion of X; nucl. of solitary tract
	GSA	External ear	Superior ganglion of X; spinal nucl. of V
Accessory (XI)	SVE	Mm. of larynx and pharynx (with X)	Nucleus ambiguus (cranial part)
	SVE or SE	Sternocleidomastoid and trapezius Mm.	Accessory nucl. (spinal part) C_1–C_5
Hypoglossal (XII)	SE	Extrinsic and intrinsic Mm. of tongue	Hypoglossal nucl.

Part of Brain Where Each Cranial Nerve Emerges and/or Enters

Nerve	Part of Brain Where Nerve Emerges/Enters
Olfactory (I)	Cerebral hemispheres (rhinencephalon — olfactory bulb)
Optic (II)	Diencephalon (laterally)
Oculomotor (III)	Midbrain (interpeduncular fossa)
Trochlear (IV)	Midbrain (just below inferior colliculi)
Trigeminal (V)	Pons (laterally)
Abducent (VI)	Pons (near midline, just above junction with medulla)
Facial (VII)	Pons — medulla junction (laterally)
Vestibulocochlear (VIII)	Pons — medulla junction (laterally)
Glossopharyngeal (IX)	Medulla (laterally — just posterior to olive)
Vagus (X)	Medulla (laterally — just posterior to olive)
Accessory (XI)	
Cranial part	Medulla (laterally — just posterior to olive)
Spinal part	C_1–C_5 spinal cord (laterally)
Hypoglossal (XII)	Medulla (near midline, between olive and pyramid)

Site of Exit from Cranium of Cranial Nerves

Nerve	Site of Exit from Cranium
Olfactory (I)	Cribriform plate, ethmoid (via olfactory foramina)
Optic (II)	Optic canal, sphenoid
Oculomotor (III)	Superior orbital fissure, sphenoid
Trochlear (IV)	Superior orbital fissure, sphenoid
Trigeminal (V)	
Ophthalmic division	Superior orbital fissure, sphenoid
Maxillary division	Foramen rotundum, sphenoid
Mandibular division	Foramen ovale, sphenoid
Abducent (VI)	Superior orbital fissure, sphenoid
Facial (VII)	Internal acoustic meatus; then: hiatus of facial canal — greater petrosal N.; petrotympanic fissure — chorda tympani N.; stylomastoid foramen — facial N. itself
Vestibulocochlear (VIII)	Internal acoustic meatus (does not leave skull)
Glossopharyngeal (IX)	Jugular foramen (except lesser petrosal N.)
Vagus (X)	Jugular foramen, temporal and occipital
Accessory (XI)	Jugular foramen, temporal and occipital
Hypoglossal (XII)	Hypoglossal canal, occipital

Note: The internal acoustic meatus, the hiatus of the facial canal, the petrotympanic fissure, and the stylomastoid foramen are all part of the temporal bone.

Rapid Neurological Evaluation of Cranial Nerve Function

Nerve	Test	Normal Finding
Olfactory (I)	Apply simple odors (e.g., peppermint, coffee) to one nostril at a time	Correct identification of the odor
Optic (II)	Visual acuity using standard eye chart	Correct identification of letters
	Visual fields using a confrontation test	No visual field defects
	Ophthalmoscopic examination	Normal fundus
Oculomotor (III) (parasympathetic component)	Flash light in one eye at a time	Ipsilateral (direct light reflex) and contralateral (consensual light reflex) pupils constrict
Oculomotor (III), trochlear (IV), and abducent (VI)	Ask person to follow your finger while you move it to the right and left, up and down, and obliquely	Both eyes follow finger in parallel (conjugate deviation)
Trigeminal (V)	Feel the two masseter muscles as person bites down; have person open his/her mouth	Equal contraction of masseters and no deviation of mandible
	Test tactile or pain sensation for all three divisions	Normal sensory perception from entire face
	Jaw jerk and corneal reflexes	
Facial (VII)	Ask person to wrinkle forehead, close eyes, show teeth	Normal execution of the movements
	Apply a small amount of sugar or salt to the anterior two-thirds of the tongue	Correct identification of the substance
Vestibulocochlear (VIII)	Hearing acuity using a watch or a whisper	Normal and bilaterally symmetrical hearing
	Rinne test (tuning fork on mastoid process, etc.)	Air conduction greater than bone conduction
	Weber test (tuning fork on center of forehead)	Heard in both ears equally
	Otoscopic examination	Normal tympanic membrane

Nerve	Test	Normal Finding
Glossopharyngeal (IX)	Touch pharynx with cotton applicator	Gagging (normal gag reflex)
Vagus (X)	Ask person to say "ah"	Both sides of soft palate contract and uvula remains in the midline
	Listen to person talk	Lack of hoarseness
Accessory (XI)	Ask person to turn his/her head to each side and shrug his/her shoulders while you resist the movements	Strong contractions of the sternocleidomastoid and trapezius muscles
Hypoglossal (XII)	Ask person to protrude his/her tongue fully	Tongue protrudes in the midline

The peripheral nervous system consists of (a) the cranial nerves, (b) the spinal nerves, and (c) the peripheral portion of the autonomic nervous system. These three morphological subdivisions are not independent functionally, but combine and communicate with each other to supply both the somatic and the visceral parts of the body with both afferent and efferent fibers.

The Cranial Nerves

The 12 pairs of cranial nerves are attached to the base of the brain (see Figures 56–63) and pass from the cranial cavity into the face and neck through various openings, or foramina, in the skull. The cranial nerves are presented in chart form on the preceding pages. What these charts do not tell you is where the nerves are located in the body. This you will learn as you study the atlas in Part IV, illustrations in other books, and cadaver specimens of gross anatomy and neuroanatomy. In the first chart, the functional components of each of the cranial nerves are listed in the order of their clinical and physiological importance.

The Spinal Nerves

The spinal nerves arise from the spinal cord within the vertebral canal and pass out through the intervertebral foramina. The 31 pairs of spinal nerves are grouped as follows: 8 cervical, 12 thoracic, 5 lumbar, 5 sacral, and 1 coccygeal. The first cervical nerve leaves the vertebral canal by passing between the occipital bone and the atlas; the eighth cervical nerve leaves between the seventh cervical and the first thoracic vertebrae; and the rest of the nerves exit below their respective vertebrae (e.g., the twelfth thoracic nerve exits between the twelfth thoracic and first lumbar vertebrae).

Each spinal nerve is formed by the union of the *dorsal* and *ventral roots* that emerge from each spinal cord segment. It is this joining of the sensory fibers of the dorsal root and the motor fibers of the ventral root that forms the basis for the mixed nature (i.e., containing SE, GSA, GVE, and GVA fibers) of the spinal nerve and its subsequent branches (Figure 1). Just after the spinal nerve passes through its intervertebral foramen, it ends by dividing into a *dorsal ramus* and a *ventral ramus* (Figure 1).

Dorsal rami of spinal nerves. The *dorsal rami* of the spinal nerves are smaller than the ventral rami. After they arise from the spinal nerves, they course posteriorly and, with a few exceptions, divide into *medial* and *lateral branches* which segmentally supply the deep back muscles and the skin of the posterior aspect of the head, neck, and trunk.

Ventral rami of spinal nerves. The *ventral rami* of the spinal nerves supply the anterior and lateral parts of the trunk and all parts of the upper and lower limbs (skin and muscles). In the thoracic region they remain independent and segmental in nature, but in the cervical, lumbar, and sacral regions they unite near their origins to form the *cervical, brachial, lumbar,* and *sacral plexuses.* As mentioned previously, the dorsal and ventral rami contain all four of the components of a typical spinal nerve (Figure 1).

Peripheral nerve fibers can be classified on the basis of several parameters such as conduction velocity of the action potential or nerve impulse, diameter of the myelin sheath, and nerve fiber diameter. Generally speaking, the larger the nerve fiber diameter, the faster the conduction velocity. Motor and sensory neurons of different sizes are associated with specific functional modalities, and these will be presented in detail in Part II.

Two classification systems are currently in use. The first system is based on the conduction velocities of both motor and sensory nerve fibers and divides nerve fibers into three groups: A, B, and C. The second system includes only sensory fibers and consists of four groups: I, II, III, and IV. This system is based primarily on nerve fiber diameter. These two classification systems are summarized in the following table.

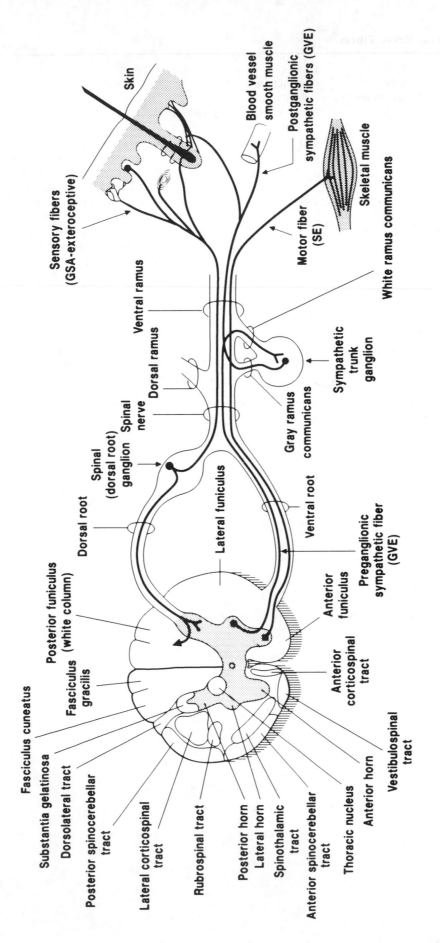

Figure 1 Schematic cross section through the upper thoracic spinal cord, illustrating the main tracts and nuclei of the spinal cord and the components of a typical spinal nerve (*no GVA neuron is shown*)

Classification of Peripheral Nerve Fibers

Sensory and Motor Fibers	Sensory Fibers	Largest Fiber Diameter (μm)	Fastest Conduction Velocity (meters/sec)	Function	
Aα	Ia	22	120	Motor:	Alpha motor neurons of lamina IX, innervating extrafusal muscle fibers
				Sensory:	The primary afferents of neuromuscular spindles (anulospiral endings)
Aα	Ib	22	120	Sensory:	Neurotendinous spindles
Aβ	II	13	70	Sensory:	The secondary afferents of neuromuscular spindles (flower spray endings), touch and pressure receptors, and pacinian corpuscles (vibratory sensors)
Aγ		8	40	Motor:	Gamma motor neurons of lamina IX, innervating intrafusal fibers (neuromuscular spindles)
Aδ	III	5	15	Sensory:	Pain and temperature fibers
B		3	14	Motor:	Preganglionic autonomic fibers
				Sensory:	Visceral afferent fibers
C	IV	1	2	Motor:	Postganglionic autonomic fibers
				Sensory:	Unmyelinated pain and temperature fibers

Part Two
Functional Neuroanatomy of the Major Sensory and Motor Pathways

Introduction

Before considering the functional neuroanatomical pathways in this section, it might be helpful to review two additional concepts that will be referred to in the pathway outlines. These are the internal organization of the spinal cord gray matter and the correlation of areas of functional localization with the cytoarchitectonic map of the cerebral cortex.

Architecture of the Spinal Cord Gray Matter

Neurons of the spinal cord gray matter are arranged in longitudinal columns according to similarity in appearance and function. In transverse section these cell columns appear as layers or laminae. This laminar scheme, as described by Rexed, is more useful in functionally organizing the gray matter than the older method of giving separate names to each of the cell columns (or nuclei). However, a few of the latter are worthy of continued use, and these will be mentioned in association with the laminae in which they reside. The laminae are numbered by Roman numerals, beginning at the tip of the posterior horn and moving anteriorly into the anterior horn (Figure 2).

Lamina I is a thin layer of neurons capping the posterior horn. It receives some pain and temperature afferent fibers from the dorsal roots and contributes some fibers to the contralateral *spinothalamic tract.*

Figure 2   Composite spinal cord section with nuclei on the right and laminae on the left

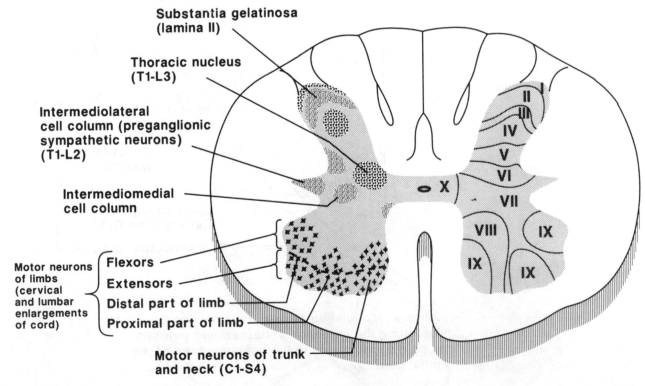

Substantia gelatinosa (lamina II)

Thoracic nucleus (T1-L3)

Intermediolateral cell column (preganglionic sympathetic neurons) (T1-L2)

Intermediomedial cell column

Motor neurons of limbs (cervical and lumbar enlargements of cord)
- Flexors
- Extensors
- Distal part of limb
- Proximal part of limb

Motor neurons of trunk and neck (C1-S4)

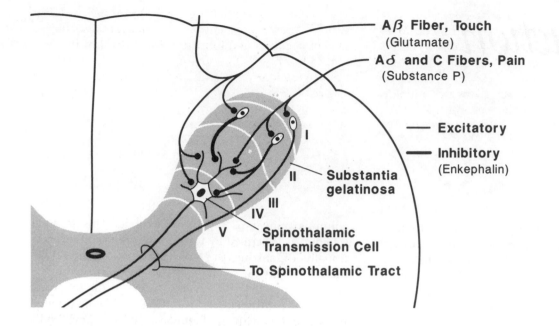

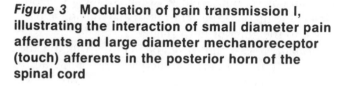

Figure 3 Modulation of pain transmission I, illustrating the interaction of small diameter pain afferents and large diameter mechanoreceptor (touch) afferents in the posterior horn of the spinal cord

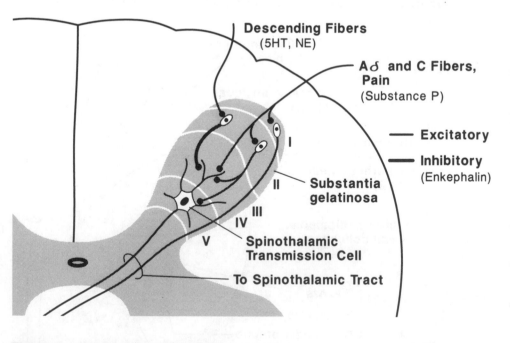

Figure 4 Modulation of pain transmission II, illustrating the influence of descending neurons on pain transmission in the posterior horn of the spinal cord

Lamina II corresponds to the *substantia gelatinosa*. It receives considerable input relating to pain, both from the dorsal root afferents and descending pathways from the nucleus raphe magnus of the medullary reticular formation. Therefore, a modulating function concerning pain perception occurs here involving multiple neurotransmitters (serotonin, norepinephrine, substance P, and enkephalin) as well as an interaction with mechanoreceptor neurons (Figures 3 and 4). Substantia gelatinosa neurons do not contribute to the ascending pain pathways directly but synapse with cells in laminae I, IV, and V.

Laminae III and *IV* are similar to lamina II, but receive larger numbers of dorsal root pain, temperature, and touch afferents. These layers are penetrated by the dendrites of the large neurons in lamina V that give rise to the fibers of the contralateral spinothalamic tract. In the upper cervical spinal cord, laminae I through IV become continuous with the inferior end of the *spinal nucleus* of the *trigeminal nerve* (*V*).

Lamina V receives dorsal root afferent fibers and interneurons from laminae II, III, and IV. Axons of these cells are the main source of the contralateral ascending pain, temperature, and light touch pathway (the *spinothalamic tract*). This lamina also receives many descending fibers from the corticospinal and rubrospinal tracts.

Lamina VI is present mainly in the cervical and lumbosacral enlargements. It receives proprioceptive input from muscles.

Lamina VII contains several important nuclei as well as many interneurons. The *intermediolateral cell column* occupies and forms the *lateral horn* of the gray matter from T_1 to L_2 and consists of the cell bodies of preganglionic sympathetic neurons. The *intermediomedial cell column* is present throughout the spinal cord and receives visceral afferent fibers. The *thoracic nucleus* (formerly known as the nucleus dorsalis or Clarke's column) is present from T_1 to L_3 and receives proprioceptive afferent fibers from neuromuscular and neurotendinous spindles. Axons of these cells form the ipsilateral *posterior spinocerebellar tract*. The *sacral parasympathetic nucleus* is present from S_2 to S_4 and consists of preganglionic parasympathetic neurons.

Lamina VIII receives descending fibers from the vestibulospinal and reticulospinal tracts involved with muscle tone, postural adjustments, and reflexes. These cells project, both ipsilaterally and contralaterally, to laminae VII and IX.

Lamina IX consists of groups (nuclei) of somatic efferent neurons whose axons leave the spinal cord in the ventral roots to supply skeletal muscles. The more medial nuclei supply the muscles of the trunk and are present at all spinal cord levels. The lateral nuclei supply the limb muscles and are present only in the cervical and lumbosacral enlargements. Both alpha and gamma motor neurons are located here.

Lamina X surrounds the central canal and is composed of decussating axons, neuroglia, and interneurons.

Cytoarchitectonic Map of the Cerebral Cortex

Figures 5 and 6 represent the lateral and medial surfaces of the brain with the most important and most commonly used cytoarchitectonic areas indicated by their numbers. The cytoarchitectonic map utilized is that of Brodmann, which is the most widely used system for correlating structural regions of the cortex with areas of functional localization. The areas indicated in Figures 5 and 6 are those referred to in the pathway outlines that follow.

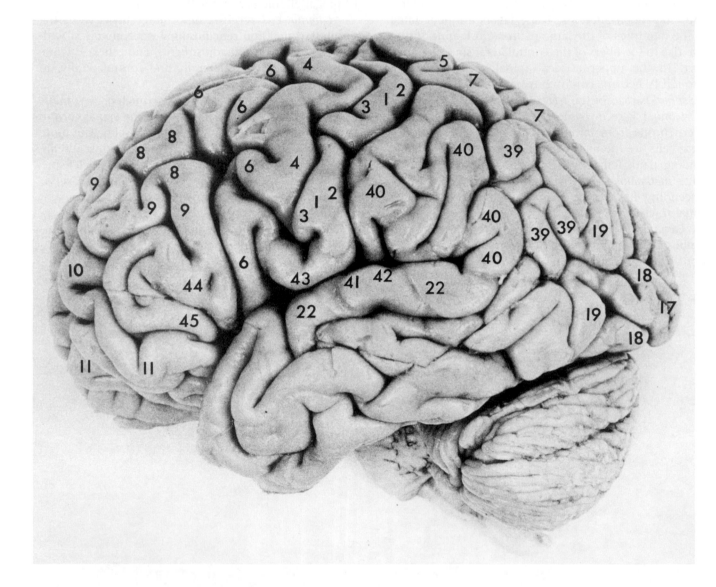

Figure 5 **Cytoarchitectonic map of the cerebral cortex, lateral view of left cerebral hemisphere**

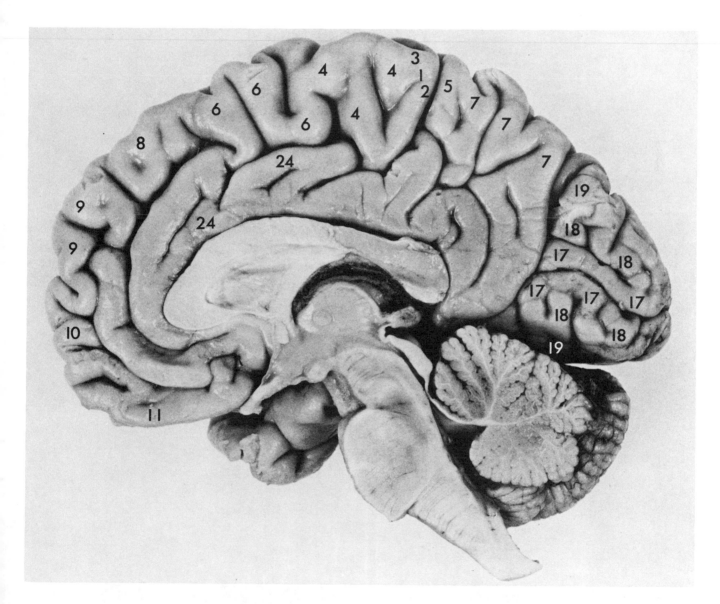

Figure 6 Cytoarchitectonic map of the cerebral cortex, medial view of right cerebral hemisphere. Median section

General Somatic Afferent Pathways

GENERAL SOMATIC AFFERENTS FROM THE BODY

Pain, Temperature, and Light (Crude) Touch
(Figures 3, 4, and 7)

1. Receptors
   a. Free nerve endings — for pain, temperature, and touch
   b. Tactile discs (Merkel) — for touch and pressure
   c. Peritrichial endings (around hair follicles) — for touch
2. Peripheral processes of pseudounipolar cell bodies (dendrites)
   a. Thinly myelinated fibers (Aδ and C — pain and temperature) and intermediately myelinated fibers (Aβ — light touch) in peripheral nerves
   b. Converge on the spinal nerves
   c. Enter the dorsal roots of the spinal nerves
3. Cell bodies of the first-order neurons
   a. Small pseudounipolar cell bodies in the spinal (dorsal root) ganglia (pain and temperature)
   b. Medium-sized pseudounipolar cell bodies in the spinal ganglia (light touch)
4. Central processes of pseudounipolar cell bodies (axons)
   a. Pain and temperature fibers
      (1) Enter the spinal cord through the lateral division of the dorsal root
      (2) Enter the *dorsolateral tract* (Lissauer)
      (3) Ascend or descend for a total of one to three segments, sending collaterals into the posterior horn all along the way
   b. Light touch fibers
      (1) Enter the spinal cord through the medial division of the dorsal root
5. First synapse (i.e., location of the second-order neuron cell bodies)
   a. Pain and temperature fibers
      (1) Marginal layer (lamina I) of the posterior horn of the spinal cord
      (2) Substantia gelatinosa (lamina II) of the posterior horn
      (3) Neurons whose cell bodies are in lamina V of the posterior horn
      (4) The substantia gelatinosa receives considerable input concerning pain from dorsal root afferents and descending pathways from the nucleus raphe magnus of the medullary reticular formation. Therefore, a modulation of pain information occurs in the substantia gelatinosa involving multiple neurotransmitters (serotonin, norepinephrine, substance P, and enkephalin) as well as an interaction with mechanoreceptor neurons (Figures 3 and 4). Substantia gelatinosa neurons do not contribute to the ascending pain pathways directly, but synapse with cells in laminae I and V. These neurons, in turn, constitute the "second-order neurons" whose axons are the main source of the contralateral ascending pain (and temperature) pathways.
   b. Light touch fibers
      (1) Posterior horn of the spinal cord, mainly neurons whose cell bodies are in lamina V
6. Course of axons of the second-order neurons
   a. Cross to the contralateral side of the cord through the white commissure while ascending about one segment
   b. Enter the *spinothalamic tract* (and spinoreticular and spinotectal tracts) in the anterolateral quad-

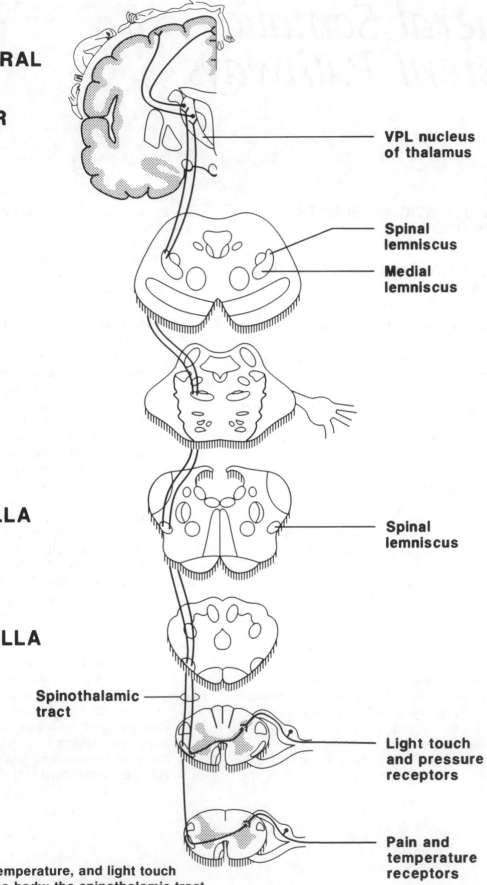

CEREBRAL CORTEX POSTCENTRAL GYRUS

POSTERIOR LIMB OF INTERNAL CAPSULE

VPL nucleus of thalamus

MIDBRAIN

Spinal lemniscus

Medial lemniscus

MID-PONS

MID-MEDULLA

Spinal lemniscus

LOW MEDULLA

Spinothalamic tract

C₇

Light touch and pressure receptors

L₄

Pain and temperature receptors

Figure 7 Pain, temperature, and light touch pathways from the body: the spinothalamic tract

rant of the spinal cord. This pathway is sometimes referred to as the *anterolateral system*

   c. Ascend in the cord to the medulla

   d. Ascend through the lateral field of the brain stem as the *spinal lemniscus*

   e. At midbrain levels, the spinal lemniscus comes to lie at the posterolateral tip of the medial lemniscus

7. Second synapse (i.e., location of the third-order neuron cell bodies)

   a. Ventral posterolateral nucleus (VPL nucleus) of the thalamus

8. Course of axons of the third-order neurons

   a. Enter the posterior limb of the internal capsule

   b. Pass through the corona radiata

   c. End in the postcentral gyrus (somesthetic cortex) of the parietal lobe of the cerebral cortex — areas 3, 1, and 2

Discriminative (Fine) Touch and Pressure (Two-Point Tactile Discrimination, Tactile Localization, Graphesthesia), Conscious Proprioception (Joint Position Sense, Kinesthesis), Vibratory Sense, and Stereognosis
(Figure 8)

1. Receptors

   a. Meissner's corpuscles — for touch

   b. Peritrichial endings — for touch

   c. Tactile discs (Merkel) — for touch and pressure

   d. Free nerve endings — for touch and conscious proprioception

   e. Pacinian corpuscles — for touch, pressure, vibration, and conscious proprioception

2. Peripheral processes of pseudounipolar cell bodies (dendrites)

   a. Intermediately myelinated fibers ($A\beta$) in peripheral nerves

   b. Converge on the spinal nerves

   c. Enter the dorsal roots of the spinal nerves

3. Cell bodies of the first-order neurons

   a. Medium-sized pseudounipolar cell bodies in the spinal ganglia

4. Central processes of pseudounipolar cell bodies (axons)

   a. Enter the spinal cord through the medial division of the dorsal root

   b. Enter the *fasciculus gracilis* (if below the T_6 level of the cord) or the *fasciculus cuneatus* (if above the T_6 level of the cord) in the posterior funiculus ipsilaterally (i.e., without crossing the midline)

   c. Ascend in the posterior funiculus to the medulla

5. First synapse

   a. Nucleus gracilis of the medulla — for fibers entering the cord below T_6 and ascending in the fasciculus gracilis

   b. Nucleus cuneatus of the medulla — for fibers entering the cord above T_6 and ascending in the fasciculus cuneatus

6. Course of axons of the second-order neurons

   a. Form the *internal arcuate fibers*

   b. Cross to the contralateral side of the medulla in the lemniscal decussation

   c. Enter the *medial lemniscus,* which is located just posterior to the pyramids of the medulla at this level

     (1) The cuneate part of the medial lemniscus is posterior to the gracile part as the medial lemniscus is formed

   d. Ascend in the brain stem, with the gracile part slowly moving laterally, then posteriorly, so that by the time the medial lemniscus reaches the midbrain, the gracile part is posterolateral to the cuneate part (other tracts have come to lie next to the medial lemniscus by this time also)

7. Second synapse

   a. VPL nucleus of the thalamus

8. Course of axons of the third-order neurons

   a. Enter the posterior limb of the internal capsule

   b. End in the postcentral gyrus (somesthetic cortex) of the parietal lobe of the cerebral cortex — areas 3, 1, and 2

Note: The traditional view of the function and organization of the posterior column pathways, as presented above, has been expanded and modified in recent years. Although the basic outline and concepts are still useful in an organizational sense for the beginning stu-

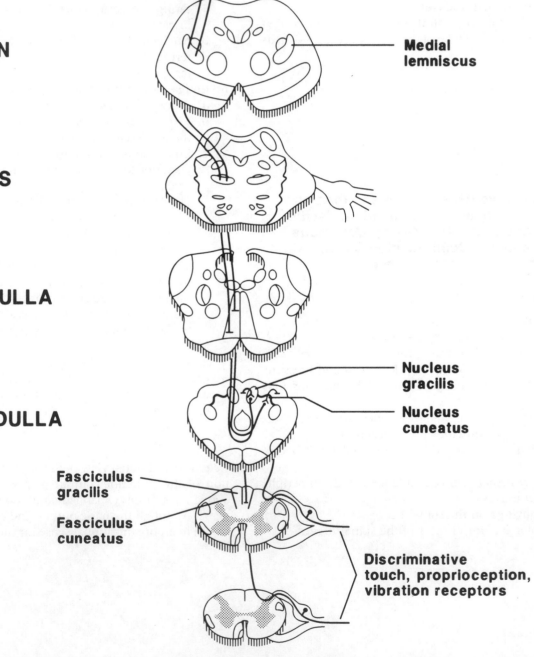

CEREBRAL CORTEX POSTCENTRAL GYRUS

POSTERIOR LIMB OF INTERNAL CAPSULE

VPL nucleus of thalamus

MIDBRAIN

Medial lemniscus

MID-PONS

MID-MEDULLA

Nucleus gracilis

LOW MEDULLA

Nucleus cuneatus

Fasciculus gracilis

C₇

Fasciculus cuneatus

Discriminative touch, proprioception, vibration receptors

L₄

Figure 8 Discriminative touch, proprioception, and vibration pathways from the body: the fasciculi gracilis and cuneatus

dent and practicing clinician, the reader should realize that this sensory system, like all of the pathways presented in this section, is more complex than originally presumed. The major modifications can be enumerated as follows:

(1) Passive sensory stimuli (touch, pressure, vibration, two-point discrimination, tactile localization) are transmitted in multiple parallel pathways (spinothalamic tract, spinocervical tract, postsynaptic or second-order neurons in the posterior columns) even though the fasciculi gracilis and cuneatus may be the most important.

(2) The sensory stimuli uniquely transmitted by the posterior columns are those concerned with temporal as well as spatial qualities (e.g., perceiving changes in stimuli over time) and those requiring active manipulation or exploration by the digits. Graphesthesia and stereognosis are examples of these types of sensory modalities.

(3) Posterior column sensations also play an important role in the performance of complex motor acts by feeding back sensory information from neuromuscular spindles, joint receptors, and cutaneous receptors to the sensorimotor cortex.

(4) It now appears that rapidly adapting joint receptors are concerned mainly with transmitting information concerning *joint movement*. These impulses probably utilize the traditional posterior column pathways (as presented above) from both the upper and lower limbs.

(5) However, the conscious perception of steady-state or static *joint position* is mediated by slowly adapting, tonically active, neuromuscular spindle receptors. The pathways mediating static joint position (as well as joint movement) from the upper limb follow the traditional fasciculus cuneatus pathway as presented above.

From the lower limb, this information is carried in the fasciculus gracilis up to the upper lumbar and lower thoracic levels of the spinal cord, where synaptic contact is made with second-order neuron cell bodies in the thoracic nucleus. The second-order neurons send their axons into the ipsilateral *posterior spinocerebellar tract*, which ascends to the medulla [and eventually passes into the cerebellum via the inferior cerebellar peduncle as part of the *unconscious proprioception* system (see *Spinocerebellar Connections: Input, p. 57*)]. In the lower medulla, fibers in the posterior spinocerebellar tract concerned with *conscious proprioception* (joint position sense) from the lower limb pass into a small nucleus adjacent to the nucleus gracilis, *nucleus Z*, and synapse with its cell bodies. Those cell bodies send their axons into the contralateral medial lemniscus and, from there, to the VPL nucleus of the thalamus.

GENERAL SOMATIC AFFERENTS FROM THE FACE

Pain, Temperature, and Light (Crude) Touch *(Figure 9)*

1. Receptors
   a. Free nerve endings
   b. Tactile discs (Merkel)
   c. Peritrichial endings
2. Peripheral processes of pseudounipolar cell bodies (dendrites)
   a. Thinly (Aδ and C) and intermediately (Aβ) myelinated fibers in the three divisions of the trigeminal nerve (V), the facial nerve (VII), the glossopharyngeal nerve (IX), and the vagus nerve (X)
3. Cell bodies of the first-order neurons
   a. Small and medium-sized pseudounipolar cell bodies in the trigeminal and geniculate ganglia and the superior ganglia of IX and X
4. Central processes of pseudounipolar cell bodies (axons)
   a. Enter the brain stem at the appropriate level for each nerve (i.e., pons or medulla)
   b. Turn inferiorly and enter the *spinal tract of the trigeminal nerve (V)* ipsilaterally
   c. Descend in the tract through the lower pons, medulla, and into the upper segments of the cervical spinal cord (C_2–C_4)

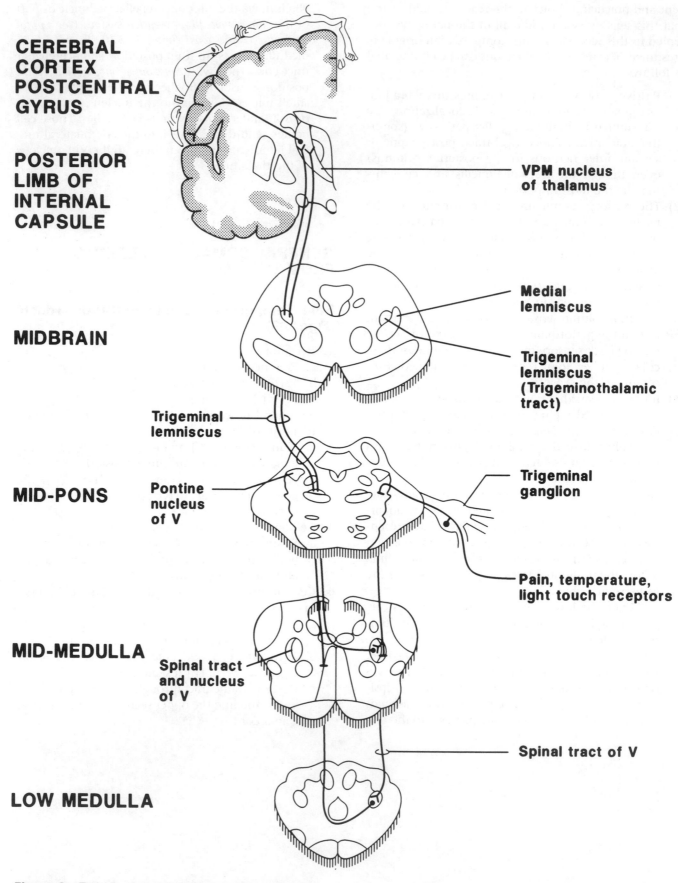

CEREBRAL CORTEX POSTCENTRAL GYRUS

POSTERIOR LIMB OF INTERNAL CAPSULE

MIDBRAIN

MID-PONS

MID-MEDULLA

LOW MEDULLA

VPM nucleus of thalamus

Medial lemniscus

Trigeminal lemniscus (Trigeminothalamic tract)

Trigeminal ganglion

Pain, temperature, light touch receptors

Trigeminal lemniscus

Pontine nucleus of V

Spinal tract and nucleus of V

Spinal tract of V

Figure 9 Pain and temperature pathways from the face: the trigeminal lemniscus

5. First synapse
   a. Spinal nucleus of the trigeminal nerve (V), all along its length
6. Course of axons of the second-order neurons
   a. Cross to the contralateral side of the brain stem
   b. Enter the *trigeminal lemniscus* (trigeminothalamic tract), which lies next to the medial lemniscus
   c. Ascend through the brain stem in this tract in association with the medial lemniscus
7. Second synapse
   a. Ventral posteromedial nucleus (VPM nucleus) of the thalamus
8. Course of axons of the third-order neurons
   a. Enter the posterior limb of the internal capsule
   b. Pass through the corona radiata
   c. End in the "face area" of the postcentral gyrus (somesthetic cortex) of the parietal lobe of the cerebral cortex — areas 3, 1, and 2

Discriminative (Fine) Touch and Pressure *(Figure 10)*

1. Receptors
   a. Meissner's corpuscles
   b. Peritrichial endings
   c. Tactile discs (Merkel)
   d. Free nerve endings
   e. Pacinian corpuscles
2. Peripheral processes of pseudounipolar cell bodies (dendrites)
   a. Intermediately myelinated fibers (Aβ) in the three divisions of the trigeminal nerve (V)
3. Cell bodies of the first-order neurons
   a. Medium-sized pseudounipolar cell bodies in the trigeminal ganglion
4. Central processes of pseudounipolar cell bodies (axons)
   a. Enter the pons through the sensory root of the trigeminal nerve (V)
5. First synapse
   a. Pontine nucleus of the trigeminal nerve (V) in the mid-pons
6. Course of axons of the second-order neurons
   a. Most fibers cross to the contralateral side of the pons and enter the *trigeminal lemniscus* (trigeminothalamic tract)
      (1) These fibers come to lie in close association with the medial lemniscus
      (2) They ascend through the brain stem along with the medial lemniscus
   b. A small number of fibers remain uncrossed

7. Second synapse
   a. VPM nucleus of the thalamus
8. Course of axons of the third-order neurons
   a. Enter the posterior limb of the internal capsule
   b. Pass through the corona radiata
   c. End in the "face area" of the postcentral gyrus (somesthetic cortex) of the parietal lobe of the cerebral cortex — areas 3, 1, and 2

Conscious and Unconscious Proprioception

1. Receptors
   a. Free nerve endings (in joint capsules, ligaments, etc.) — conscious proprioception
   b. Pacinian corpuscles — conscious proprioception
   c. Neurotendinous spindles — unconscious proprioception
   d. Neuromuscular spindles (anulospiral and flower-spray endings) in muscles of mastication (possibly facial, extraocular, and tongue muscles, too) — unconscious and conscious proprioception
2. Peripheral processes of pseudounipolar cell bodies (dendrites)
   a. Heavily (Aα, Ia and Ib) and intermediately (Aβ) myelinated fibers in the three divisions of the trigeminal nerve (V) (mainly the mandibular division)
   b. Pass through the trigeminal ganglion without synapsing
   c. Enter the pons through the motor and sensory roots of the trigeminal nerve (V)
   d. Turn upward and enter the *mesencephalic tract of V* on the ipsilateral side
3. Cell bodies of the first-order neurons
   a. Large and medium-sized pseudounipolar cell bodies in the *mesencephalic nucleus of V* in the upper pons and midbrain
4. Central processes of pseudounipolar cell bodies (axons)
   a. Pass from the mesencephalic nucleus of V back into the mesencephalic tract of V ipsilaterally
   b. Descend in the tract
5. First synapse
   a. Pontine nucleus of V — fibers concerned with conscious proprioception
   b. Motor nucleus of V in the mid-pons — for motor reflexes such as the jaw jerk
   c. Probably the facial nucleus and other motor nuclei of cranial nerves as well
   d. Reticular formation

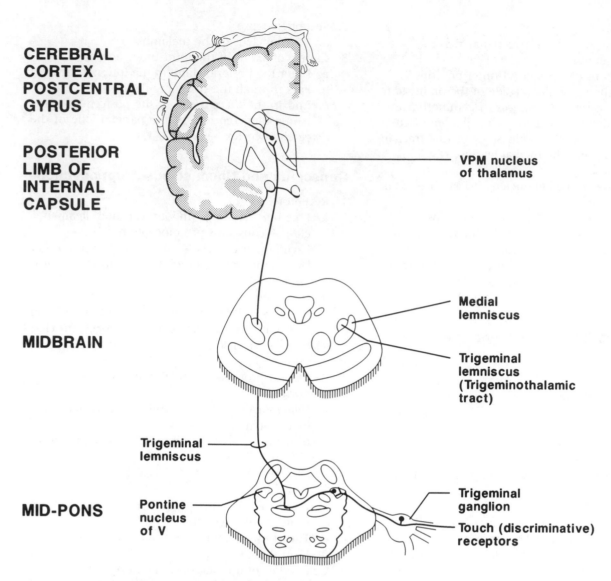

CEREBRAL CORTEX POSTCENTRAL GYRUS

POSTERIOR LIMB OF INTERNAL CAPSULE

VPM nucleus of thalamus

MIDBRAIN

Medial lemniscus

Trigeminal lemniscus (Trigeminothalamic tract)

Trigeminal lemniscus

MID-PONS

Pontine nucleus of V

Trigeminal ganglion

Touch (discriminative) receptors

Figure 10 **Discriminative touch pathways from the face: the trigeminal lemniscus**

6. Course of axons of the second-order neurons
   a. Fibers from the pontine nucleus of V ascend through the brain stem in the *dorsal trigeminal tract*
   b. Fibers from stretch receptors probably pass into the cerebellum
7. Second synapse
   a. VPM nucleus of the thalamus — fibers for conscious proprioception
8. Course of axons of the third-order neurons
   a. Enter the posterior limb of the internal capsule
   b. Pass through the corona radiata
   c. End in the "face area" of the postcentral gyrus (somesthetic cortex) of the parietal lobe of the cerebral cortex — areas 3, 1, and 2

Special Visceral Afferent Pathways

Taste
(Figure 11)

1. Receptors
   a. Neuroepithelial cells of the taste buds located on the fungiform and circumvallate papillae of the tongue and the epiglottis
2. Peripheral processes of pseudounipolar cell bodies (dendrites)
   a. Special visceral afferent components of the facial (VII), glossopharyngeal (IX), and vagus (X) nerves
   b. Run toward the brain stem in their respective nerves
3. Cell bodies of the first-order neurons
   a. Pseudounipolar cell bodies in the geniculate ganglion of VII — fibers from the anterior two-thirds of the tongue

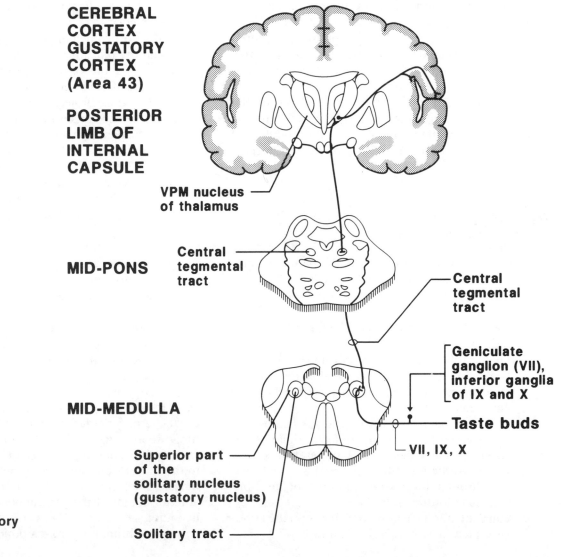

CEREBRAL CORTEX GUSTATORY CORTEX (Area 43)

POSTERIOR LIMB OF INTERNAL CAPSULE

VPM nucleus of thalamus

MID-PONS

Central tegmental tract

Central tegmental tract

Geniculate ganglion (VII), inferior ganglia of IX and X

Taste buds

MID-MEDULLA

VII, IX, X

Superior part of the solitary nucleus (gustatory nucleus)

Solitary tract

Figure 11 Gustatory (taste) pathways

b. Pseudounipolar cell bodies in the inferior ganglion of IX — fibers from the posterior third of the tongue (including the circumvallate papillae)

c. Pseudounipolar cell bodies in the inferior ganglion of X — fibers from the epiglottic region of the tongue and the epiglottis

4. Central processes of pseudounipolar cell bodies (axons)
   a. Enter the pons and the medulla through the roots of the facial, glossopharyngeal, and vagus nerves
   b. Enter the *solitary tract* (tractus solitarius)

5. First synapse
   a. Superior part of the nucleus of the solitary tract (gustatory nucleus) at or near the levels of the respective nerves

6. Course of axons of the second-order neurons
   a. Enter the ipsilateral *central tegmental tract*
   b. Ascend through the brain stem in this tract

7. Second synapse
   a. VPM nucleus of the thalamus

8. Course of axons of the third-order neurons
   a. Enter the posterior limb of the internal capsule
   b. Pass through the corona radiata
   c. End in the lowermost part of the .postcentral gyrus (parietal operculum) of the cerebral cortex (area 43) and in the insular cortex adjacent to area 43
      (1) May also end in the cortex of the frontal operculum, adjacent insular cortex, and the posterolateral quadrant of the orbitofrontal cortex (also see olfactory pathways concerning this area)

Smell
(Figure 12)

1. Receptors
   a. Olfactory hairs at the ends of the peripheral processes of the bipolar olfactory cells

2. Peripheral processes of bipolar cell bodies (dendrites)
   a. The peripheral processes of the bipolar olfactory cells

3. Cell bodies of the first-order neurons
   a. The cell bodies of the bipolar olfactory cells located in the olfactory region (or epithelium) of the nasal cavity

4. Central processes of bipolar cell bodies (axons)
   a. Delicate central processes (olfactory fila) of the olfactory cells collect into bundles [collectively known as the olfactory nerve (I)]
   b. Pass through the olfactory foramina of the cribriform plate of the ethmoid
   c. Enter the olfactory bulb, which lies on the cribriform plate

5. First synapse
   a. Mitral and tufted cells of the olfactory bulb

6. Course of axons of the second-order neurons
   a. Enter the *olfactory tract*
   b. The olfactory tract divides into the *medial* and *lateral olfactory striae*
   c. Medial olfactory stria
      (1) Fibers entering this tract have their cell bodies in the *anterior olfactory nucleus*, a group of cell bodies scattered along the olfactory tract posterior to the olfactory bulb
      (2) These fibers reach the opposite olfactory bulb through the anterior commissure
   d. Lateral olfactory stria
      (1) Fibers entering this tract terminate in the anterior perforated substance (olfactory tubercle), corticomedial part of the amygdaloid body, the uncus, and the most anterior portion of the parahippocampal gyrus.

7. Second synapse
   a. The anterior portion of the parahippocampal gyrus and the uncus (which receive fibers from the lateral olfactory stria) constitute the *primary olfactory cortex*
   b. The corticomedial part of the amygdaloid body and the olfactory tubercle

8. Course of axons of the third-order neurons
   a. Axons of cell bodies located in the primary olfactory cortex project to the *entorhinal cortex* (area 28), which constitutes a major portion of the anterior parahippocampal gyrus. The entorhinal cortex is regarded as the *secondary olfactory cortex*.
      (1) Efferent fibers from the entorhinal cortex project via the *uncinate fasciculus* to the posterolateral quadrant of the orbitofrontal cortex, an area that may be important in olfactory discrimination (and taste sensation).
      (2) The entorhinal cortex also projects to the hippocampus, providing an olfactory input into memory function.
   b. The amygdaloid body and the olfactory tubercle project to the hypothalamus, the septal area, and regions of the brain stem. These connections are thought to be involved in autonomic, emotional, and endocrine manifestations of the perception of odors.

Note: In discussing the olfactory system many authors use the term *pyriform lobe* or *cortex*. Exactly which structures are included in the definition of this entity varies from author to author. Some equate the pyriform lobe to the uncus alone, whereas others include the uncus, the lateral olfactory stria, the entorhinal cortex, and the anterior extent of the parahippocampal gyrus in their definition of the area. To avoid confusion I have used descriptive human neuroanatomical terms rather than

Figure 12   Olfactory (smell) pathways

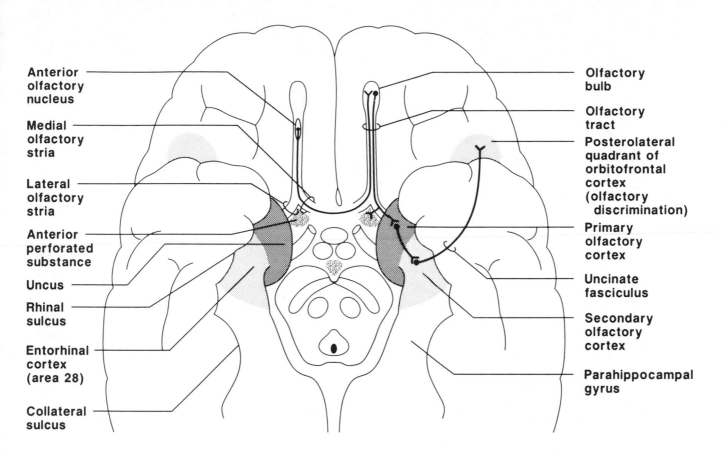

Anterior olfactory nucleus

Medial olfactory stria

Lateral olfactory stria

Anterior perforated substance

Uncus

Rhinal sulcus

Entorhinal cortex (area 28)

Collateral sulcus

Olfactory bulb

Olfactory tract

Posterolateral quadrant of orbitofrontal cortex (olfactory discrimination)

Primary olfactory cortex

Uncinate fasciculus

Secondary olfactory cortex

Parahippocampal gyrus

the comparative term, pyriform lobe, when discussing these pathways.

Unlike other sensory systems, the olfactory pathway to the primary (and secondary) olfactory cortex is not relayed through the thalamus. However, there is an olfactory pathway from the primary olfactory cortex to the *medial dorsal nucleus of the thalamus* that projects to the posterolateral orbitofrontal cortex. This appears to be a parallel pathway related to the function of olfactory discrimination (see entorhinal cortex projection pathways above).

Special Somatic Afferent Pathways

Vision
(Figures 13 and 14)

1. Receptors
   a. Rods (for black and white vision and vision in the dark) and cones (for color vision and sharp vision) located in the retina of the eyeball
2. Peripheral processes of bipolar cell bodies (dendrites)
   a. The rods and cones have short central processes that synapse with the dendrites of the bipolar cells of the retina
3. Cell bodies of the first-order neurons
   a. Bipolar cells located in the retina
4. Central processes of bipolar cell bodies (axons)
   a. Remain in the retina
5. First synapse
   a. This synapse occurs between the axons of the bipolar cells and the dendrites or cell bodies of the ganglion cells of the retina
6. Course of axons of the second-order neurons
   a. Converge on the optic disc (blind spot) of the eyeball
   b. Leave the eyeball to enter the optic nerve (II)
   c. Leave the orbit through the optic canal of the sphenoid
   d. The two optic nerves come together at the *optic chiasma*
      (1) In the optic chiasma the fibers whose (ganglion) cell bodies are located in the medial half of each eyeball cross to the contralateral side, whereas the fibers from the lateral half of the retina remain uncrossed
   e. After this partial crossing in the chiasma, the fibers enter the *optic tracts*, which course around the lateral sides of the diencephalon and end in the lateral geniculate bodies
7. Second synapse
   a. Lateral geniculate body of the thalamus
8. Course of axons of the third-order neurons
   a. Enter the *geniculocalcarine tract* (or *optic radiations*)
   b. Pass through the sublentiform and retrolentiform parts of the internal capsule
   c. End in the visual cortex on the superior and inferior lips of the calcarine sulcus (on the medial side of the occipital lobe and around the occipital pole onto the most posterior aspect of the lateral surface of the occipital lobe) — area 17
   d. Areas 18 and 19, comprising the rest of the medial and lateral surfaces of the occipital lobe, are called the *visual association areas* and must be intact if you are to interpret what you see

Figure 13 Visual pathways

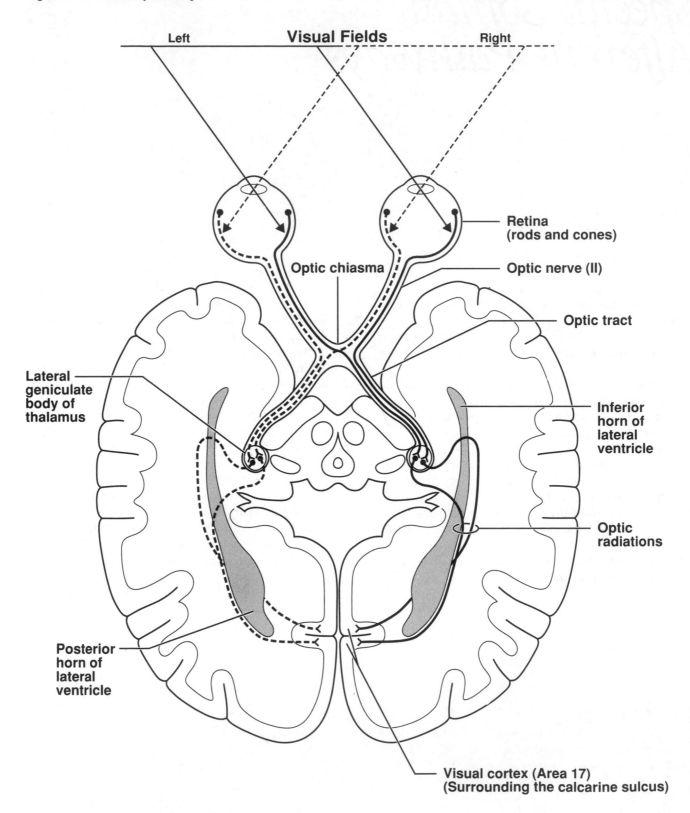

Visual Fields

Left   Right

Retina (rods and cones)

Optic chiasma

Optic nerve (II)

Optic tract

Lateral geniculate body of thalamus

Inferior horn of lateral ventricle

Optic radiations

Posterior horn of lateral ventricle

Visual cortex (Area 17) (Surrounding the calcarine sulcus)

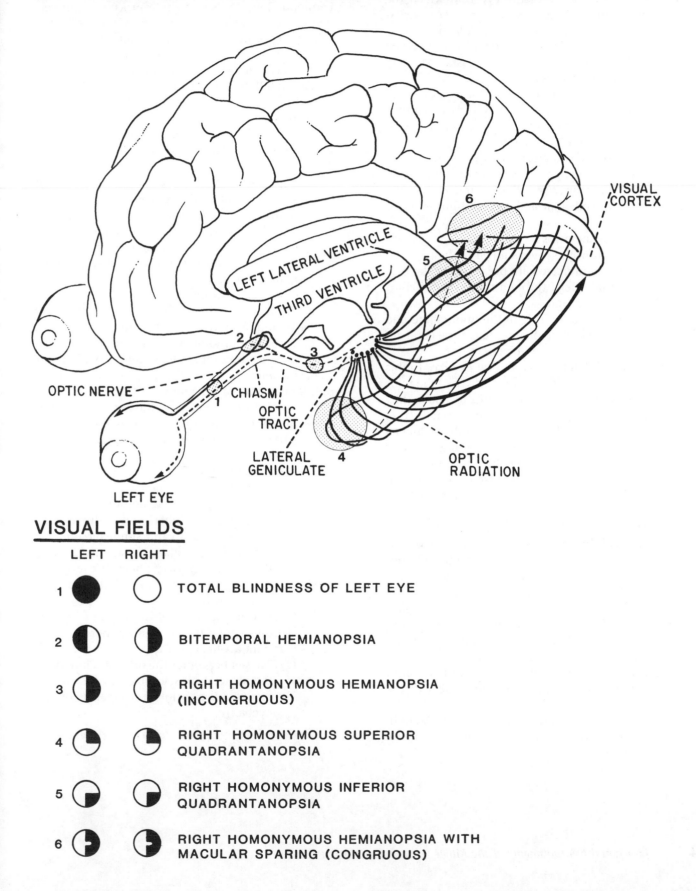

Figure 14 The visual pathways of the left side of the brain as seen with the left hemisphere removed except for the left lateral ventricle and the left visual cortex. Note the relationship of the optic radiation to the lateral ventricle. The visual field deficits produced by lesions 1 to 6 are indicated below the drawing

VISUAL FIELDS

LEFT   RIGHT

1   TOTAL BLINDNESS OF LEFT EYE

2   BITEMPORAL HEMIANOPSIA

3   RIGHT HOMONYMOUS HEMIANOPSIA (INCONGRUOUS)

4   RIGHT HOMONYMOUS SUPERIOR QUADRANTANOPSIA

5   RIGHT HOMONYMOUS INFERIOR QUADRANTANOPSIA

6   RIGHT HOMONYMOUS HEMIANOPSIA WITH MACULAR SPARING (CONGRUOUS)

Visual (Parasympathetic) Reflexes

A. Pupillary light reflexes (Figure 15)

When a light is shined into one eye, both pupils constrict. The response of the eye into which the light was shined is termed a *direct light reflex*, whereas the response of the contralateral eye is called a *consensual light reflex*. The pathway involved in both of these reflexes utilizes the visual pathway just presented at its onset.

1. Afferent limb of the reflex
   a. Fibers from the ganglion cells of the stimulated retina enter the optic nerve, optic chiasma, and both optic tracts
   b. Some of these fibers, rather than synapsing in the lateral geniculate body, enter the *brachium of the superior colliculus* and end in the superior collicular and pretectal nuclei of the midbrain
2. Internuncial neurons
   a. Axons from the pretectal cell bodies
      (1) Communicate with the contralateral pretectal nuclei through the posterior commissure, and
      (2) Course anteriorly in the midbrain to end in the ipsilateral and the contralateral accessory oculomotor nucleus
   b. Note that light shined in one eye has, to this point in the reflex pathway, crossed the midline (at least partially) in three locations (i.e., the optic chiasma, the posterior commissure, and the tract between the pretectal nuclei and the accessory oculomotor nuclei). This crossing is the basis for the consensual light reflex, whereas the uncrossed fibers at each of these locations form the basis for the direct light reflex.
3. Efferent limb of the reflex
   a. Axons from the cells of the accessory oculomotor nucleus enter the ipsilateral oculomotor nerve as parasympathetic preganglionics (GVE) and run with the nerve into the orbit
   b. In the orbit these fibers enter the ciliary ganglion (through the oculomotor root of the ciliary ganglion) and synapse with the postganglionic neurons of the ganglion
   c. Axons of these cells run forward (as short ciliary nerves) and pierce the sclera of the eyeball
   d. These fibers eventually innervate the smooth muscle fibers of the sphincter pupillae muscle of the iris

B. Accommodation

When a person who is looking at something off in the distance quickly focuses on an object nearby, a complex reaction called *accommodation* occurs. Accommodation consists of three processes: convergence of the eyeballs, constriction of the pupil, and thickening of the lens for near vision.

There are two theories concerning the mechanism of accommodation. One theory is that accommodation follows convergence, being initiated by it; the other holds that accommodation occurs simultaneously with convergence. The latter theory will be explained here, but the pathways are not too different for the former theory.

1. Afferent limb of the reflex
   a. Light on the retina evokes impulses that travel by way of the regular visual pathways to area 17 of the cortex
   b. Impulses probably also reach the superior colliculus (and pretectal nuclei) through the brachium of the superior colliculus (as in the light reflex above)
2. Internuncial neurons
   a. From area 17, impulses travel to areas 18 and 19 and, from there, to the superior colliculus
   b. Tecto-oculomotor fibers travel to the accessory oculomotor nucleus and the oculomotor nucleus
3. Efferent limb of the reflex
   a. Fibers from the cells of the accessory oculomotor nucleus enter the oculomotor nerve (III) as parasympathetic preganglionics (GVE)
      (1) These fibers enter the orbit and synapse in the ciliary ganglion with parasympathetic postganglionic neurons
      (2) Postganglionic fibers enter the eyeball and distribute to the sphincter pupillae muscle (for pupillary constriction) and to the smooth muscle fibers of the ciliary muscle (for thickening of the lens for near vision)
   b. Fibers from the cells of the oculomotor nucleus also enter the oculomotor nerve [as somatic motor fibers (SE)]
      (1) These fibers enter the orbit and innervate the skeletal muscle fibers of the medial rectus muscle (for convergence of the eyeball)

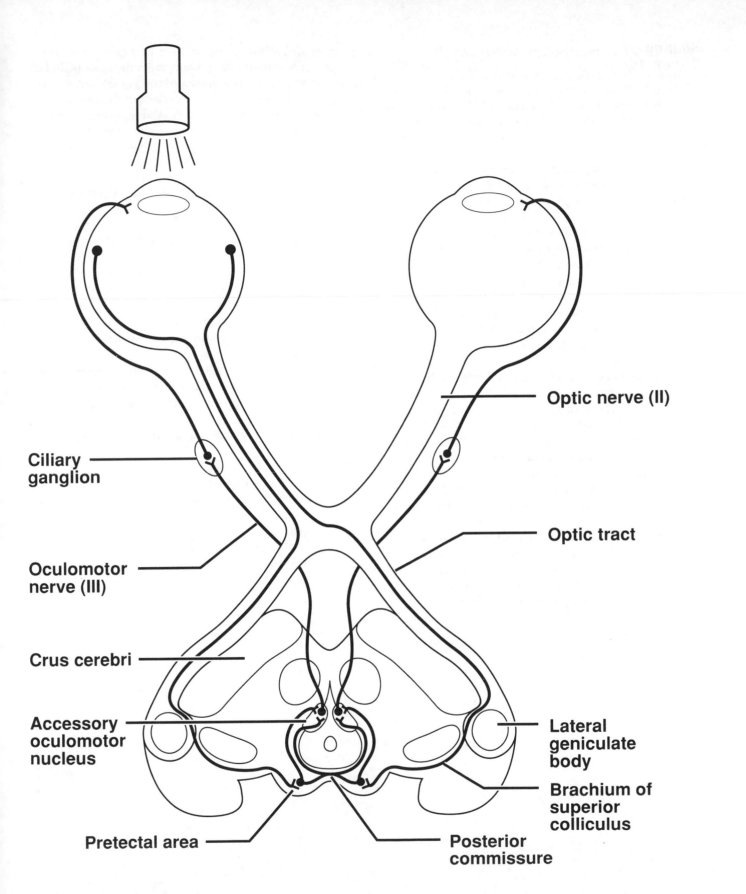

Ciliary ganglion

Oculomotor nerve (III)

Crus cerebri

Accessory oculomotor nucleus

Optic nerve (II)

Optic tract

Lateral geniculate body

Brachium of superior colliculus

Pretectal area

Posterior commissure

Figure 15 **Pupillary light reflex pathways**

Hearing
(Figure 16)

1. Receptors
   a. Inner and outer hair cells of the spiral organ located in the cochlear duct of the cochlea
2. Peripheral processes of bipolar cell bodies (dendrites)
   a. Short peripheral processes of the bipolar cells of the cochlear (spiral) ganglion
3. Cell bodies of the first-order neurons
   a. Bipolar cells of the cochlear (spiral) ganglion located in the modiolus of the cochlea
4. Central processes of bipolar cell bodies (axons)
   a. Converge to form the cochlear part of the vestibulocochlear nerve (VIII)
   b. Leave the petrous part of the temporal bone through the internal acoustic meatus
   c. Enter the pons–medulla junction by way of the vestibulocochlear nerve (VIII)
5. First synapse
   a. Dorsal and ventral cochlear nuclei of the lower pons–upper medulla
6. Course of axons of the second-order neurons
   a. Most (but not all) of the fibers cross to the contralateral side of the pons in the trapezoid body (and other parts of the pons)
   b. Enter the *lateral lemniscus*
   c. The lateral lemniscus ascends through the brain stem and ends (mainly) in the inferior colliculus
   d. As the lateral lemniscus is formed and ascends through the brain stem, fibers leave and enter it — going to and coming from the nuclei of the trapezoid body, the superior olivary nucleus, and the nucleus of the lateral lemniscus
   e. In addition to those fibers that cross in the trapezoid body, some fibers cross the midline in between the two nuclei of the lateral lemnisci (in the upper pons), others cross in the commissure of the inferior colliculi, and still others remain uncrossed and ascend in the ipsilateral lateral lemniscus
      (1) Therefore, in some cases these second-order neurons may be third- or fourth-order neurons by the time they reach the inferior colliculus
7. Second synapse
   a. Mainly in the inferior colliculus of the midbrain
   b. As mentioned above, also in the nuclei of the trapezoid body, the superior olivary nucleus, and the nucleus of the lateral lemniscus
8. Course of axons of the third-order neurons
   a. Enter the *brachium of the inferior colliculus*
   b. Ascend to enter the medial geniculate body
9. Third synapse
   a. Medial geniculate body of the thalamus
10. Course of axons of the fourth-order neurons
    a. Enter the *geniculocortical fibers* (or *auditory radiations*)
    b. Pass through the sublentiform part of the internal capsule
    c. End in the primary auditory cortex (area 41) and the secondary auditory cortex (area 42) on the transverse temporal gyri of the temporal lobe
    d. Area 22, on the superior temporal gyrus of the temporal lobe, is the *auditory association area* and must be intact if you are to interpret what you hear

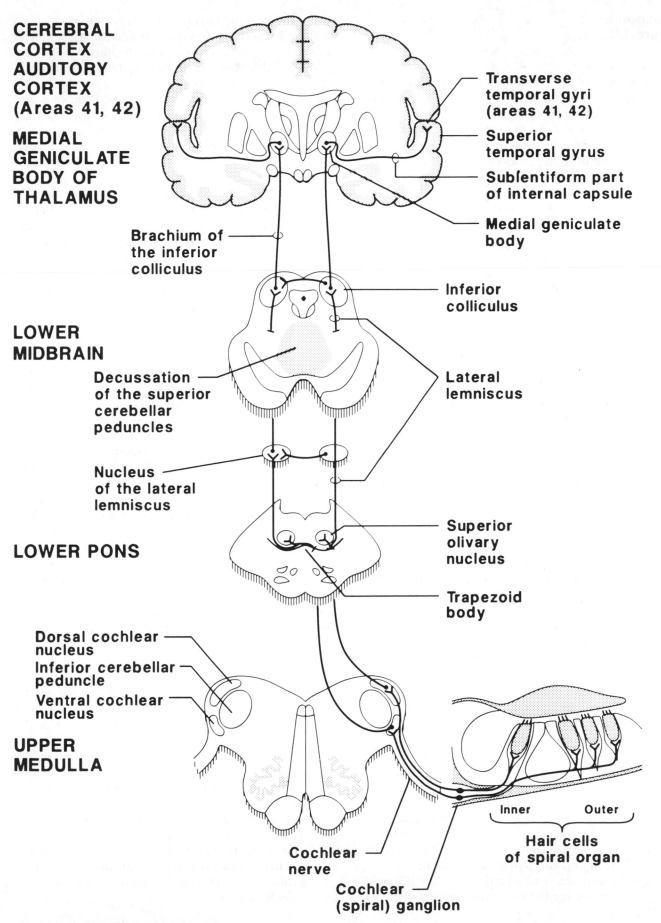

CEREBRAL CORTEX AUDITORY CORTEX (Areas 41, 42)

MEDIAL GENICULATE BODY OF THALAMUS

Transverse temporal gyri (areas 41, 42)

Superior temporal gyrus

Sublentiform part of internal capsule

Medial geniculate body

Brachium of the inferior colliculus

Inferior colliculus

LOWER MIDBRAIN

Decussation of the superior cerebellar peduncles

Lateral lemniscus

Nucleus of the lateral lemniscus

LOWER PONS

Superior olivary nucleus

Trapezoid body

Dorsal cochlear nucleus

Inferior cerebellar peduncle

Ventral cochlear nucleus

UPPER MEDULLA

Inner

Outer

Hair cells of spiral organ

Cochlear nerve

Cochlear (spiral) ganglion

Figure 16 **Auditory pathways**

Equilibrium
(Figure 17)

1. Receptors
   a. Hair cells of the crista ampullaris located in the ampulla of each semicircular duct — for dynamic equilibrium (angular acceleration)
   b. Hair cells of the macula utriculi and the macula sacculi located in the utricle and the saccule of the vestibule of the inner ear — for static equilibrium (changes in gravitational forces, linear acceleration, and the position of the head in space)
2. Peripheral processes of bipolar cell bodies (dendrites)
   a. Short peripheral processes of the bipolar cells of the vestibular ganglion
3. Cell bodies of the first-order neurons
   a. Bipolar cells of the vestibular ganglion located in the internal acoustic meatus
4. Central processes of bipolar cell bodies (axons)
   a. Form the vestibular part of the vestibulocochlear nerve (VIII)
   b. Leave the petrous part of the temporal bone through the internal acoustic meatus
   c. Enter the pons–medulla junction by way of the vestibulocochlear nerve (VIII)
   d. *Some* (not most) of the fibers enter the ipsilateral side of the cerebellum and end in the cortex of the uvula, flocculus, and nodulus (flocculonodular lobe, vestibulocerebellum, archicerebellum)
5. First synapse
   a. Superior, lateral, medial, and inferior vestibular nuclei of the upper medulla–lower pons
6. Course of axons of the second-order neurons
   a. Fibers from the inferior and medial vestibular nuclei enter the cerebellum and end in the nodulus, flocculus, uvula, and the fastigial nucleus
      (1) The cortex of the vestibulocerebellum (flocculonodular lobe) and the fastigial nuclei send efferent fibers to all four vestibular nuclei (and the brain stem reticular formation) bilaterally via the inferior cerebellar peduncle
   b. Fibers from the lateral vestibular nucleus enter the *vestibulospinal tract,* which distributes throughout the length of the spinal cord ipsilaterally, facilitating reflex activity and extensor muscle tone
      (1) This tract helps control body movements in response to vestibular stimuli
   c. Fibers from all of the vestibular nuclei enter the *medial longitudinal fasciculus* (MLF). These fibers are both crossed and uncrossed, and many split into ascending and descending branches.
      (1) Descending vestibular fibers in the MLF arise from the medial vestibular nucleus (perhaps also the lateral and inferior nuclei)
         (a) They descend through the medulla and enter the anterior funiculus of spinal cord
         (b) They distribute only to the cervical spinal cord
         (c) This tract helps control head and arm movements in response to vestibular stimuli
      (2) Ascending vestibular fibers in the MLF arise from all the vestibular nuclei. They mainly project to the nuclei of the extraocular muscles (i.e., the oculomotor, trochlear, and abducent nuclei). Thus, the main function of these fibers is to provide vestibular, and probably cerebellar, input into the functioning of the extraocular muscles. There are pathways controlling the horizontal movement of the eyes subsequent to turning the head horizontally, and the vertical movement of the eyes subsequent to turning the head vertically. Both of these pathways enable you to focus on a point as you turn your head. This represents the "vestibulo-ocular reflex (VOR)," which has also been referred to as the "nonoptic reflex eye movement system."
         (a) Vestibular neurons concerned with horizontal eye movements project to the contralateral abducent nucleus, which contains two populations of neurons (see section on *Eye Movements*). The abducent motor neurons supply the lateral rectus muscle ipsilaterally, whereas the abducent internuclear neurons project via the contralateral MLF to the medial rectus subdivision of the oculomotor nucleus.
         (b) Vestibular neurons controlling vertical eye movements project via the MLF bilaterally to the oculomotor and trochlear nuclei.
7. Vestibulo-cortical pathways
   a. Fibers from the superior, medial, and lateral vestibular nuclei project diffusely and bilaterally to the ventral posterolateral (VPL) nucleus of the thalamus
   b. VPL neurons project to various regions of the parietal lobe (areas 3, 2, and 5) and probably also to parts of the temporal lobe (superior temporal gyrus)
   c. This pathway enables you to consciously perceive vestibular sensations (movement of the head, position of the head in space, etc.). Many of the neurons in this pathway are activated by a convergence of proprioceptive, visual, and vestibular inputs.

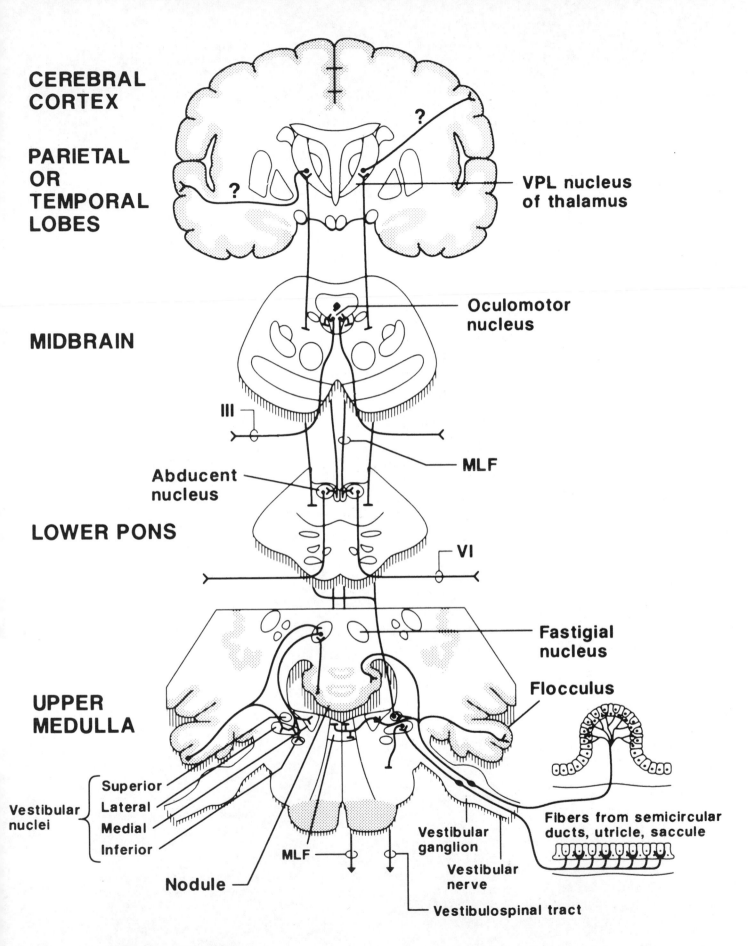

CEREBRAL CORTEX

PARIETAL OR TEMPORAL LOBES

?

?

VPL nucleus of thalamus

MIDBRAIN

Oculomotor nucleus

III

MLF

Abducent nucleus

LOWER PONS

VI

Fastigial nucleus

Flocculus

UPPER MEDULLA

Vestibular nuclei

Superior
Lateral
Medial
Inferior

MLF

Nodule

Vestibular ganglion

Vestibular nerve

Vestibulospinal tract

Fibers from semicircular ducts, utricle, saccule

Figure 17   **Vestibular pathways**

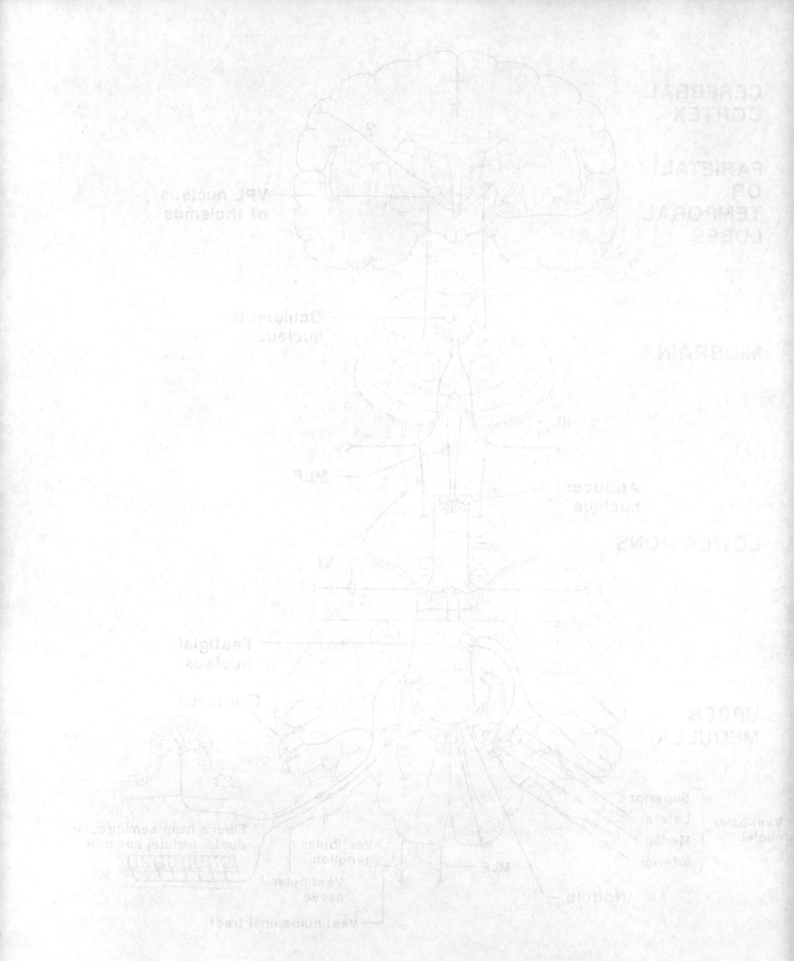

Motor Pathways

EYE MOVEMENTS

The pathways that control eye movements are varied and complex. Gay and his colleagues described five different eye movement systems: the saccadic system (for rapid, voluntary eye movements), the smooth pursuit system (for following or tracking eye movements), the vergence system (for convergence or divergence), the nonoptic reflex system (for reflex eye movements in response to vestibular or neck receptor stimuli), and the position maintenance system (for maintaining gaze fixation on a target). Leigh and Zee use the term "vestibulo-ocular reflex" (VOR) as a synonym for the nonoptic reflex system. The pathways mediating these various types of eye movement are known to variable degrees. Those pathways controlling conjugate eye movements [saccades, pursuit, and VOR (nonoptic reflexes)] are known in greater detail than those governing the vergence system and the position maintenance system. I will describe only the saccadic system and the smooth pursuit system here, because these are the systems most commonly tested clinically and the systems about which we know the most. The vestibulo-ocular reflex (VOR, nonoptic reflex) system was alluded to previously in the section on equilibrium.

The Saccadic System (Rapid Eye Movements, Voluntary Eye Movements)

Saccadic eye movements are controlled by parallel pathways involving the frontal eye fields (area 8) and the superior colliculi. The frontal eye fields, and perhaps the posterior parietal cortex (area 7), are concerned with voluntarily directing the eyes toward an object of interest, whereas the superior colliculi are involved in continuously reorienting gaze to visual stimuli. Lesions involving only one of these areas produce subtle deficits in saccadic eye movements, but damage to both areas drastically impairs ocular mobility. The details of the projections to and from the superior colliculi are less well understood than those from the frontal eye fields, and therefore only the latter will be described in this section.

There are two pathways that govern voluntary, or rapid, eye movements (saccades), one for horizontal eye movements and one for vertical eye movements. These are outlined separately below.

A. Pathway for voluntary horizontal conjugate eye movements (Figure 18)
1. Location of upper motor neuron cell bodies
   a. Motor cortex for voluntary eye movements (frontal eye field, area 8) located mainly on the middle frontal gyrus of the frontal lobe
   b. Horizontal eye movements are mediated by the contralateral frontal eye field (i.e., horizontal conjugate eye movements to the right are controlled by the left frontal lobe, and vice versa)
2. Course of axons of the upper motor neurons
   a. Fibers pass through the corona radiata
   b. Pass into the anterior limb of the internal capsule, where the pathway divides into a portion that enters the thalamus ("transthalamic pathway") and ultimately ends in the ipsilateral pretectal area, superior colliculus, and central gray substance of the midbrain
   c. The other portion of the pathway ("ventral pathway") passes through the most medial aspect of the crus cerebri of the midbrain
   d. In the upper pons, the fibers pass into the paramedian pontine reticular formation (PPRF), which is located just anterior and lateral to the MLF extending from the abducent nucleus to just inferior to the trochlear nucleus. A partial decussation occurs in the PPRF.
   e. In the PPRF, the fibers synapse with various types of neurons (burst cells, pause cells, tonic cells) involved in generating saccadic eye movements.
   f. In the lower third of the pons, the neurons of the PPRF send their axons into the ipsilateral abducent nucleus
      (1) The abducent nucleus contains two types of neurons: *abducent motor neurons* that supply the ipsilateral lateral rectus mus-

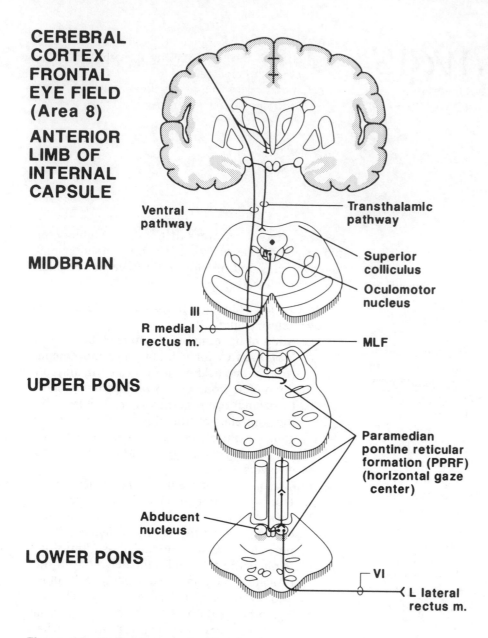

CEREBRAL CORTEX FRONTAL EYE FIELD (Area 8)

ANTERIOR LIMB OF INTERNAL CAPSULE

Ventral pathway

Transthalamic pathway

MIDBRAIN

Superior colliculus

Oculomotor nucleus

III

R medial rectus m.

MLF

UPPER PONS

Paramedian pontine reticular formation (PPRF) (horizontal gaze center)

Abducent nucleus

LOWER PONS

VI

L lateral rectus m.

Figure 18 **Pathways controlling horizontal saccadic eye movements**

cle, and *abducent internuclear neurons* that project into the contralateral MLF and ascend to synapse with the medial rectus motor neurons in the oculomotor nucleus. PPRF neurons synapse with both types of abducent neurons.

    (2) Therefore, the PPRF near the abducent nucleus plus the abducent nucleus constitute the *pontine horizontal gaze center*

3. Location of lower motor neuron cell bodies
   a. Abducent nucleus — abducent motor neurons
   b. The part of the oculomotor nucleus (contralateral to the abducent nucleus) that controls the medial rectus muscle
4. Course of axons of the lower motor neurons
   a. Enter the abducent nerve (VI) and travel with it into the orbit

   b. Enter the contralateral oculomotor nerve (III) and travel with it into the orbit
5. Structures innervated
   a. Lateral rectus muscle via the abducent nerve
   b. Contralateral medial rectus muscle via the oculomotor nerve

B. Pathway for voluntary vertical conjugate eye movements (Figure 19)
1. Location of upper motor neuron cell bodies
   a. Motor cortex for voluntary eye movements (frontal eye field, area 8) located mainly on the middle frontal gyrus of the frontal lobe
   b. Vertical eye movements are mediated by simultaneous activity of both frontal eye fields; therefore, unilateral supranuclear (upper motor neuron) lesions will not affect vertical eye movements
2. Course of axons of the upper motor neurons

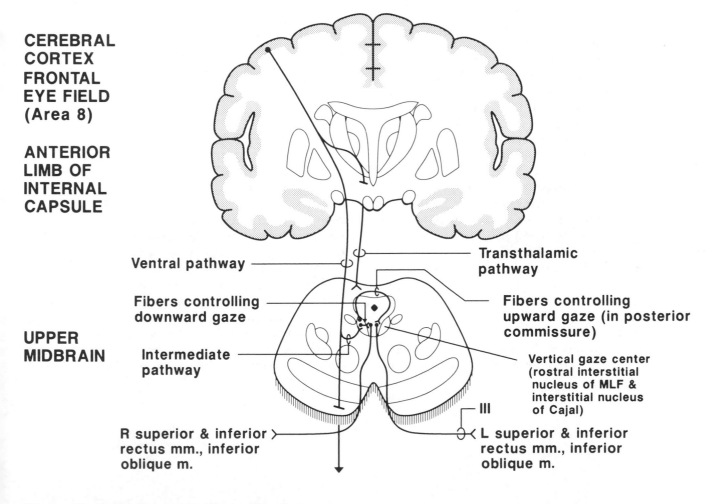

CEREBRAL CORTEX FRONTAL EYE FIELD (Area 8)

ANTERIOR LIMB OF INTERNAL CAPSULE

UPPER MIDBRAIN

Ventral pathway

Fibers controlling downward gaze

Intermediate pathway

R superior & inferior rectus mm., inferior oblique m.

Transthalamic pathway

Fibers controlling upward gaze (in posterior commissure)

Vertical gaze center (rostral interstitial nucleus of MLF & interstitial nucleus of Cajal)

III

L superior & inferior rectus mm., inferior oblique m.

Figure 19 **Pathways controlling vertical saccadic eye movements**

a. Fibers pass through the corona radiata (bilaterally)

b. Pass into the anterior limb of the internal capsule, where the pathway divides into the two portions mentioned above (i.e., the "transthalamic pathway" ending in the pretectum and superior colliculus and the "ventral pathway" passing through the crus cerebri to enter the PPRF)

c. At the diencephalon–mesencephalon junction (the pretectal region) an "intermediate pathway" forms with bilateral contributions from both the transthalamic and ventral pathways

d. In the pretectal region of the upper midbrain, this pathway sends crossed and uncrossed fibers into the *rostral interstitial nucleus* of the *MLF* and the *interstitial nucleus* (*Cajal*), which constitute the *pretectal vertical gaze center*

  (1) The pretectal vertical gaze center receives inputs from ascending projections of the vestibular nuclei and PPRF as well as the descending projections of the transthalamic and intermediate pathways from the frontal eye fields just mentioned

  (2) The neurons of the pretectal vertical gaze center project their axons bilaterally into the oculomotor and trochlear nuclei of the midbrain (the trochlear projections are not shown in Figure 19)

  (3) Projections to the elevator or upgaze subnuclei (innervating the superior rectus and inferior oblique muscles) pass above the cerebral aqueduct in the posterior commissure. Projections to the depressor or downgaze subnuclei (innervating the inferior rectus and superior oblique muscles) pass anterior to or below the cerebral aqueduct.

3. Location of lower motor neuron cell bodies

a. All parts of the oculomotor nuclei except those that innervate the medial rectus muscles

b. Trochlear nuclei

4. Course of axons of the lower motor neurons

a. Enter the oculomotor nerves (III) and travel with them into the orbits

b. Cross the midline in the tectum of the midbrain, enter the trochlear nerves (IV), and travel with them into the orbits

5. Structures innervated

a. Superior and inferior rectus muscles and the inferior oblique muscles via the oculomotor nerves

b. Superior oblique muscles via the trochlear nerves

The Smooth Pursuit System (Following, or Tracking, Eye Movements)

The pathways controlling smooth pursuit eye movements are incompletely known. It appears that the posterior parietal, anterior occipital, and perhaps posterior temporal regions of the cerebral cortex (areas 18, 19, and 7) are important in smooth pursuit movements, but the exact pathway or pathways carrying their influence to the brain stem centers for conjugate gaze are poorly understood. The cortical areas seem to project to ipsilateral pontine nuclei and perhaps pretectal nuclei. These areas, in turn, may influence smooth pursuit eye movements via projections to and from the cerebellum and other brain stem areas. Some of these brain stem pathways may be similar to those utilized in saccadic eye movements.

THE PYRAMIDAL SYSTEM

Many areas of the brain are involved in the execution of complex, coordinated motor activity. These areas include the cerebral cortex, basal nuclei, subthalamic nucleus, substantia nigra, red nucleus, brain stem reticular formation, vestibular nuclei, cerebellum, and thalamus. Obviously with so many regions of the brain involved, the control and execution of movement is very complex. In this section and the sections on the basal nuclei and cerebellum, I will attempt to simplify and organize the pathways controlling movement to facilitate your understanding of its basic components under normal conditions. In this way I hope that the clinical manifestations of dysfunction involving an individual component of the motor system will ultimately be more understandable.

In discussing the pathways controlling voluntary movement, it is useful, if not entirely accurate, to utilize a conceptual schema consisting of a two neuron chain from the cerebral cortex to the skeletal muscles. This chain begins with an *upper motor neuron* whose cell body is located in the cerebral cortex and whose axon (most often) crosses the median plane to synapse with lower motor neuron cell bodies in the cranial nerve motor nuclei or the anterior horn of the spinal cord (Figure 20).

The second neuron in the chain is the *lower motor neuron*, consisting of an *alpha motor neuron* (anterior horn cell or motor neuron in a cranial nerve nucleus) and its axon. A lower motor neuron and all of the extrafusal skeletal muscle fibers it supplies are known as a *motor unit*. *Gamma motor neurons* supply the polar regions of intrafusal muscle fibers of the neuromuscular spindle and thereby control the length and tension of the spindles, which are the receptors for the stretch reflex, unconscious proprioception, and (the joint position component of) conscious proprioception. This gamma loop is very important for the optimal functioning of the motor unit. Damage to lower motor neurons anywhere along their course (a "lower motor neuron lesion") produces a group of signs and symptoms in the muscle(s) supplied by those neurons. These signs include: (1) weakness or paralysis; (2) hypotonia or flaccidity; (3) hyporeflexia or areflexia; (4) muscular atrophy; and (5) fasciculations.

The concept of the "upper motor neuron" is clinically useful although unsatisfactory in an anatomical and physiological sense. In addition to the more direct neuronal pathways mentioned above (the corticospinal and corticonuclear tracts), the "upper motor neuron" also collectively refers to several descending pathways that ultimately influence and control (along with local and segmental reflexes) the activity of the lower motor neuron. These parallel descending pathways originate

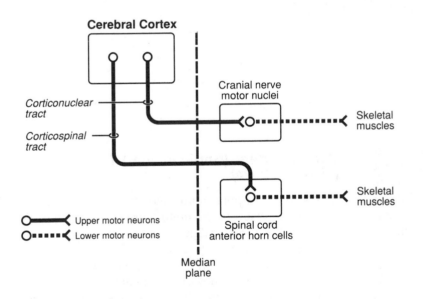

Figure 20 **The pyramidal system: two-neuron concept**

Figure 21   Concept of the "upper motor neuron"

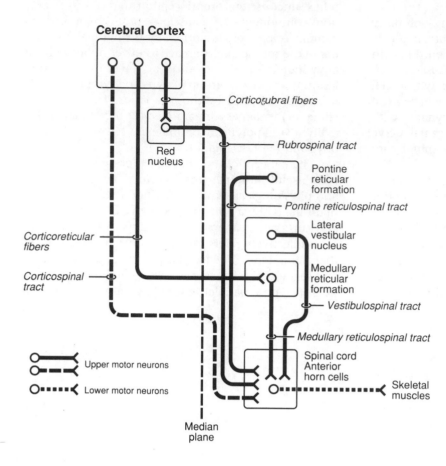

Cerebral Cortex

Corticorubral fibers

Red nucleus

Rubrospinal tract

Pontine reticular formation

Pontine reticulospinal tract

Corticoreticular fibers

Lateral vestibular nucleus

Medullary reticular formation

Corticospinal tract

Vestibulospinal tract

Medullary reticulospinal tract

Spinal cord Anterior horn cells

Skeletal muscles

Upper motor neurons

Lower motor neurons

Median plane

in areas of the brain stem such as the red nucleus (rubrospinal tract), the reticular formation of the pons and medulla (reticulospinal tracts), and the medial and lateral vestibular nuclei (MLF and vestibulospinal tract). These brain stem areas, in turn, receive afferent input from the cerebral cortex, parts of the cerebellum, and ascending sensory systems (Figure 21). "Upper motor neuron lesions" almost always damage some of these parallel pathways as well as the pyramidal system pathways. Therefore, the resulting signs and symptoms vary somewhat but usually consist of many or all of the following: (1) paralysis or weakness of voluntary movements, especially highly coordinated and skilled movements of the hand; (2) hypertonia or spasticity; (3) hyperreflexia with or without clonus; (4) absence of profound muscular atrophy or fasciculations; (5) abnormal or extensor plantar reflex — dorsiflexion or extension of the great toe and abduction of the lesser four toes when the lateral border of the sole of the foot is stimulated with a slightly pointed object; and (6) diminished or absent superficial reflexes (abdominal, cremasteric).

Corticonuclear (Corticobulbar) Tract (Figures 22–24)

1. Location of upper motor neuron cell bodies
   a. Face region of the motor cortex (area 4) located on the precentral gyrus of the frontal lobe
   b. Also areas 6, 3, 1, 2, and 5
2. Course of axons of the upper motor neurons
   a. Pass through the corona radiata
   b. Pass through the third quarter of the posterior limb of the internal capsule
   c. Pass through the medial side of the middle three-fifths of the crus cerebri of the midbrain
   d. Pass through the dispersed pyramidal tract bundles of the pons
   e. In the middle third of the pons, crossed and uncrossed fibers pass into the *motor nucleus of the trigeminal nerve* (*V*) and the nearby reticular formation
   f. In the lower third of the pons, mainly crossed (but also some uncrossed) fibers pass into the part of the *facial nucleus* that supplies the lower

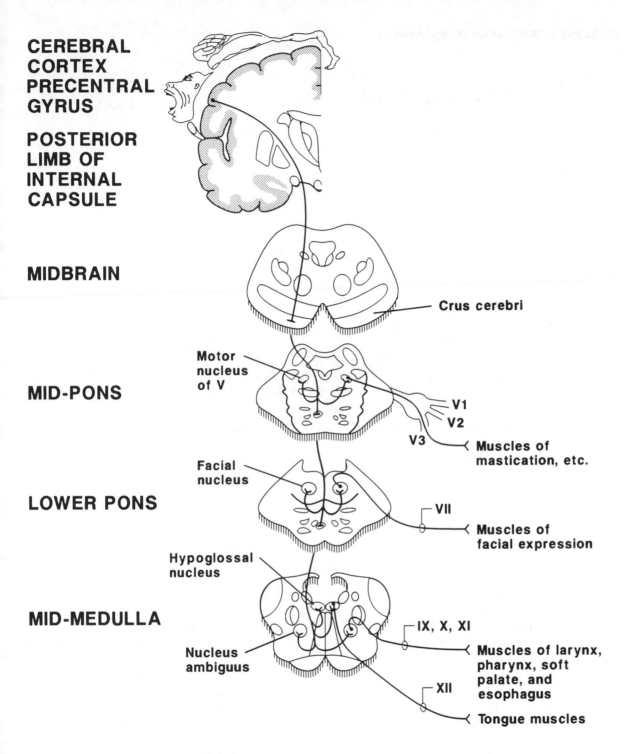

**CEREBRAL
CORTEX
PRECENTRAL
GYRUS**

**POSTERIOR
LIMB OF
INTERNAL
CAPSULE**

MIDBRAIN

Crus cerebri

MID-PONS

Motor
nucleus
of V

V1
V2
V3

Muscles of
mastication, etc.

LOWER PONS

Facial
nucleus

VII

Muscles of
facial expression

MID-MEDULLA

Hypoglossal
nucleus

IX, X, XI

Muscles of larynx,
pharynx, soft
palate, and
esophagus

Nucleus
ambiguus

XII

Tongue muscles

Figure 22   Corticonuclear (corticobulbar) tracts

Figure 23 Upper motor neuron facial weakness: new concept

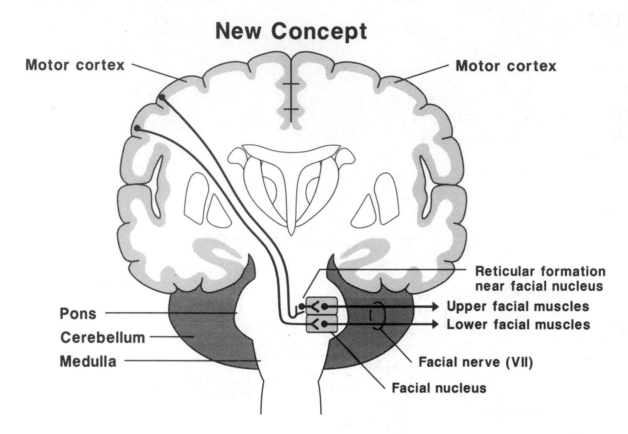

New Concept

Motor cortex

Motor cortex

Reticular formation near facial nucleus
Upper facial muscles
Lower facial muscles

Pons
Cerebellum
Medulla

Facial nerve (VII)

Facial nucleus

facial muscles and into the reticular formation near the part of the nucleus supplying the upper facial muscles

g. In the medulla, the *pyramidal tract* reunites and forms the pyramids of the medulla

h. In the medulla, crossed and uncrossed fibers pass into the *nucleus ambiguus* and surrounding reticular formation

i. In the lower medulla, crossed and uncrossed fibers pass into the *hypoglossal nucleus* and nearby reticular formation

j. Most of the axons terminate in the reticular formation near the above mentioned cranial nerve nuclei and synapse with interneurons that project into the nuclei

  (1) Axons concerned with lower facial movements synapse directly with neurons in the facial nucleus. Those concerned with upper facial movements terminate in the reticular formation near the facial nucleus and synapse with interneurons that project into the nucleus

  (2) This difference in the termination of the up-

per motor neurons forms the basis for the contralateral lower facial weakness associated with upper motor neuron lesions (Figure 23)

  (3) In the past the neuroanatomical basis for the contralateral upper motor neuron facial weakness was attributed to the presence of bilateral upper motor neuron input into the part of the facial nucleus supplying upper facial muscles, as opposed to the more vulnerable contralateral input into the part of the nucleus supplying lower facial muscles (Figure 24). Recent studies have not verified this older concept.

3. Location of lower motor neuron cell bodies

a. Motor nucleus of V

b. Facial nucleus

c. Nucleus ambiguus

d. Accessory nucleus — this is the nucleus of the spinal part of the accessory nerve (XI) that is located in the first five segments of the cervical spinal cord. These cell bodies synapse with mainly crossed upper motor neurons.

Figure 24 Upper motor neuron facial weakness: old concept

Old Concept

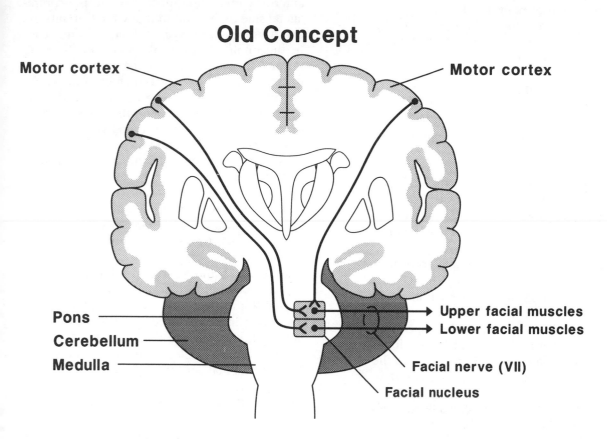

Motor cortex

Motor cortex

Pons

Cerebellum

Medulla

Upper facial muscles
Lower facial muscles

Facial nerve (VII)

Facial nucleus

e. Hypoglossal nucleus
4. Course of axons of the lower motor neurons
   a. Fibers distribute with the mandibular division of the trigeminal nerve (V)
   b. Fibers distribute with the facial nerve (VII)
   c. Fibers distribute with the glossopharyngeal nerve (IX), the vagus nerve (X), and the cranial part of the accessory nerve (XI)
   d. Fibers distribute with the spinal part of the accessory nerve (XI)
   e. Fibers distribute with the hypoglossal nerve (XII)
5. Structures innervated
   a. Muscles of mastication; tensor veli palatini, tensor tympani, mylohyoid, and anterior digastric muscles via the trigeminal nerve (mandibular division)
   b. Muscles of facial expression, stapedius, stylohyoid, and posterior digastric muscles via the facial nerve
   c. Stylopharyngeus via the glossopharyngeal nerve; muscles of the soft palate, pharynx, esophagus, and larynx via the vagus nerve (the cranial part of the accessory nerve may also supply the mus-

cles of the larynx and the pharynx)
   d. Sternocleidomastoid and trapezius muscles via the spinal part of the accessory nerve
   e. Intrinsic and extrinsic muscles of the tongue via the hypoglossal nerve
6. Function
   a. Voluntary control of rapid, finely coordinated, skilled movements of the muscle groups mentioned above
      (1) As mentioned, because the lower facial muscles are innervated monosynaptically, they are capable of more finely controlled and rapid movements than the upper facial muscles.
      (2) On the other hand, this anatomical relationship renders the lower facial muscles more vulnerable to impaired function and weakness in the event of a contralateral lesion of the upper motor neurons.

Corticospinal Tract
(Figures 25 and 26)

1. Location of upper motor neuron cell bodies
   a. Upper limb, trunk, and lower limb regions of the motor cortex (area 4) located on the precentral gyrus of the frontal lobe
   b. Also areas 6, 3, 1, 2, and 5
2. Course of axons of the upper motor neurons
   a. Enter the *corticospinal part of the pyramidal tract* [the other part of the pyramidal tract being the *corticonuclear (or corticobulbar) fibers,* outlined on the preceding pages]
   b. Pass through the corona radiata
   c. Pass through the third quarter of the posterior limb of the internal capsule
   d. Pass through the middle and lateral side of the middle three-fifths of the crus cerebri of the midbrain
   e. Pass through the dispersed pyramidal tract bundles of the pons
   f. In the medulla, the *pyramidal tract* reunites and forms the pyramids of the medulla
   g. In the low medulla, the fibers to the upper limb (first) and the lower limb (lower in the medulla) cross to the contralateral side of the body in the *pyramidal decussation* and form the *lateral corticospinal tract* of the spinal cord
      (1) 75% to 90% of the corticospinal fibers cross in the pyramidal decussation
      (2) Many of the fibers to the trunk muscles remain uncrossed and form the *anterior corticospinal tract* of the spinal cord
   h. The two corticospinal tracts then descend in the lateral and anterior funiculi of the spinal cord to the level of their synapses
   i. In the cervical cord, upper limb fibers leave the lateral corticospinal tract and pass into the gray matter of the spinal cord
   j. In the thoracic cord mainly, but also in the cervical and lumbar cords, the trunk fibers leave the anterior corticospinal tract, cross to the contralateral side of the cord in the white commissure, and pass into the gray matter of the spinal cord
   k. In the lumbar and sacral regions of the cord, lower limb fibers leave the lateral corticospinal tract and pass into the gray matter of the cord
   l. Some upper motor neurons synapse directly with the alpha motor neurons of the anterior horn of the spinal cord (in lamina IX). Others, however (as in the brain stem), synapse with internuncial neurons in lamina VII, which in turn synapse with the alpha motor neurons of the anterior horn. Still others terminate in the base of the posterior horn (laminae IV and V) and function in modulating reflex arcs and somatic sensory transmission during movement (Figure 26).
3. Location of lower motor neuron cell bodies
   a. Alpha motor neurons located in the nuclei of the medial (for trunk muscles) and lateral (for upper and lower limb muscles) divisions of the anterior horn of the spinal cord (lamina IX)
4. Course of axons of the lower motor neurons
   a. Leave the spinal cord through the ventral roots
   b. Pass into the spinal nerves
   c. Pass into the dorsal rami (only fibers to trunk muscles) and the ventral rami (upper limb, lower limb, and trunk fibers) of the spinal nerves
   d. Distribute with all of the muscular branches of the dorsal and ventral rami of the spinal nerves
5. Structures innervated
   a. Skeletal muscles of the upper and lower limbs and the trunk
6. Function
   a. Voluntary control of rapid, finely coordinated, skilled movements (especially of the hands)

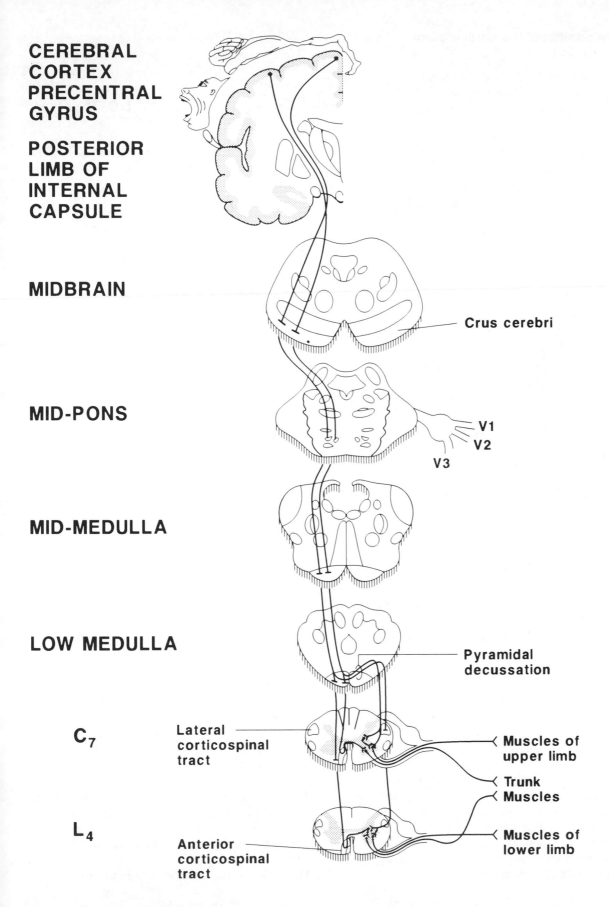

CEREBRAL CORTEX PRECENTRAL GYRUS

POSTERIOR LIMB OF INTERNAL CAPSULE

MIDBRAIN

Crus cerebri

MID-PONS

V1
V2
V3

MID-MEDULLA

LOW MEDULLA

Pyramidal decussation

C₇

Lateral corticospinal tract

Muscles of upper limb

Trunk Muscles

L₄

Anterior corticospinal tract

Muscles of lower limb

Figure 25 **Corticospinal tracts**

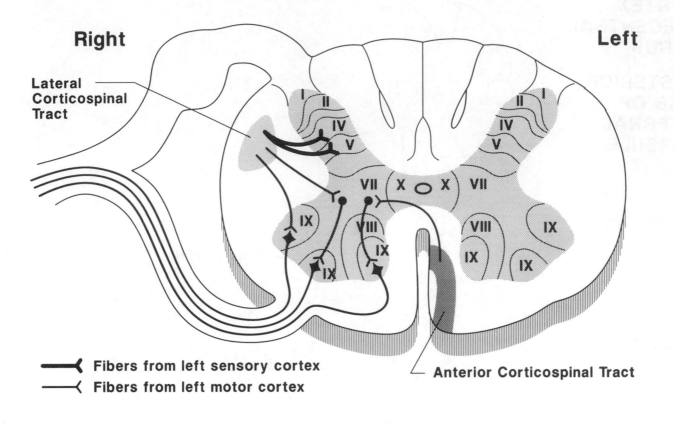

Figure 26 Termination of the corticospinal tracts

Right

Lateral Corticospinal Tract

Left

(Roman numerals I–X labeling spinal cord gray matter laminae)

═══< **Fibers from left sensory cortex**
───< **Fibers from left motor cortex**

Anterior Corticospinal Tract

CEREBELLAR CONNECTIONS

Although the cerebellum functions at an unconscious, involuntary level, it is an extremely important part of the brain with respect to motor functioning. It receives sensory input from all of the general and special senses and has efferent connections (direct or indirect) with most parts of the central nervous system. The cerebellum receives most of its afferent fibers through the inferior and middle cerebellar peduncles, whereas most of its efferent fibers leave by way of the superior and inferior cerebellar peduncles. The cerebellum is primarily concerned with three types of functional mechanisms: those that influence and maintain equilibrium, those that regulate muscle tone, and those that regulate the timing and precision (i.e., coordination) of somatic motor activity. Therefore, although there are several pathways and patterns of cerebellar connections, I will describe only the four main groups of connections by which the cerebellum exerts its influence.

Vestibular (Archicerebellar) Connections (*Figures 27–31*)

1. Input
   a. Primary (directly from the vestibulocochlear nerve) and secondary (from the vestibular nuclei) vestibular fibers enter the cerebellum through the *inferior cerebellar peduncle* and end as the mossy fibers of the archicerebellum (or *flocculonodular lobe*)
   b. The mossy fibers synapse with granule cells, which in turn synapse with Purkinje cells in the cerebellar cortex
2. Output
   a. The Purkinje cells of the archicerebellum project to the fastigial nucleus of the cerebellum
   b. The cells of the fastigial nucleus send their axons out of the cerebellum mainly through the *inferior cerebellar peduncle*
   c. These fibers end in the vestibular nuclei and

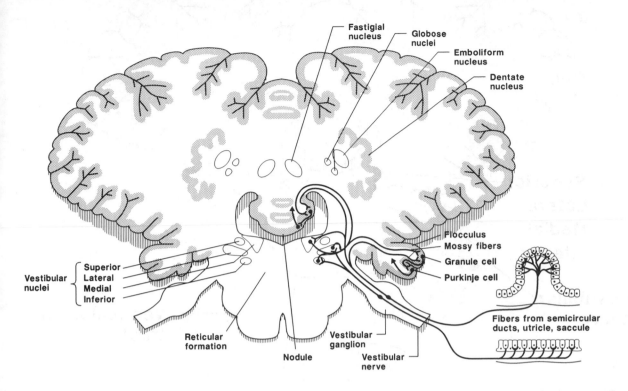

Figure 27 Vestibulocerebellar (archicerebellar) connections: vestibular input

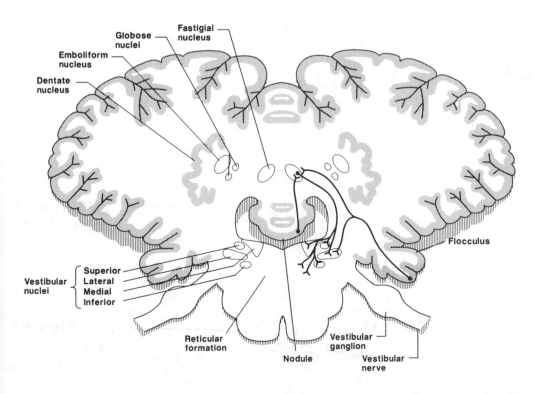

Figure 28 Vestibulocerebellar (archicerebellar) connections: cerebellar output

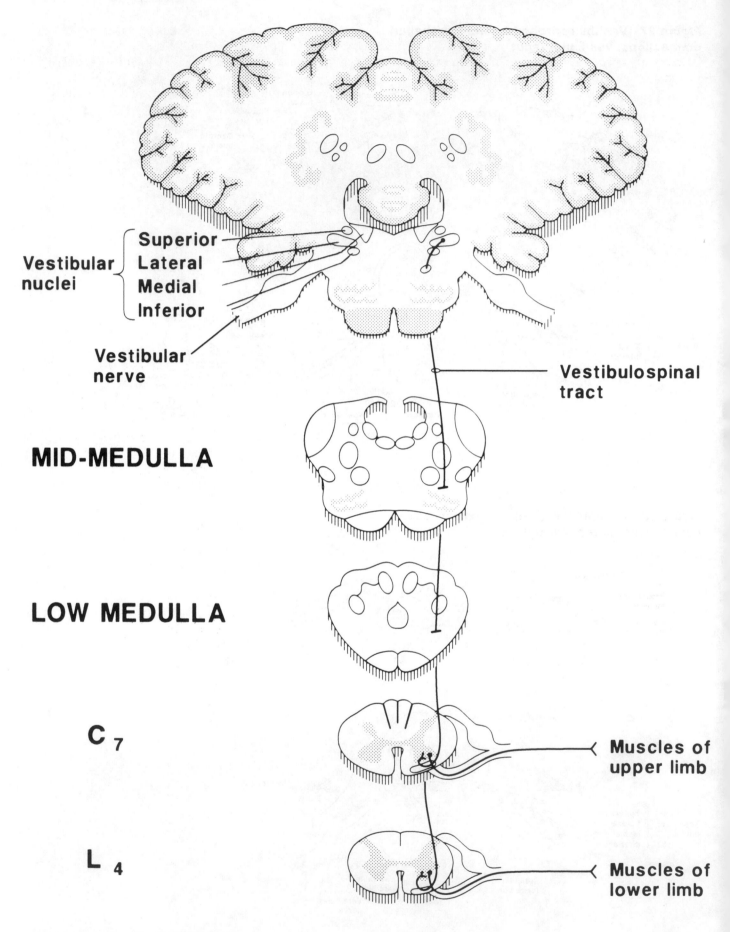

Vestibular
nuclei

Superior
Lateral
Medial
Inferior

Vestibular
nerve

Vestibulospinal
tract

MID-MEDULLA

LOW MEDULLA

C 7

L 4

Muscles of
upper limb

Muscles of
lower limb

Figure 29 **Vestibulospinal tract**

brain stem reticular formation

d. These fibers influence lower motor neurons by way of the *vestibulospinal tract,* the *recticulospinal tracts,* and the *medial longitudinal fasciculus* (MLF) (Figures 29–31).

3. Function

a. Maintenance of equilibrium

b. Regulation of the posture and balance of the trunk

c. Coordination of head, neck, and eye movements

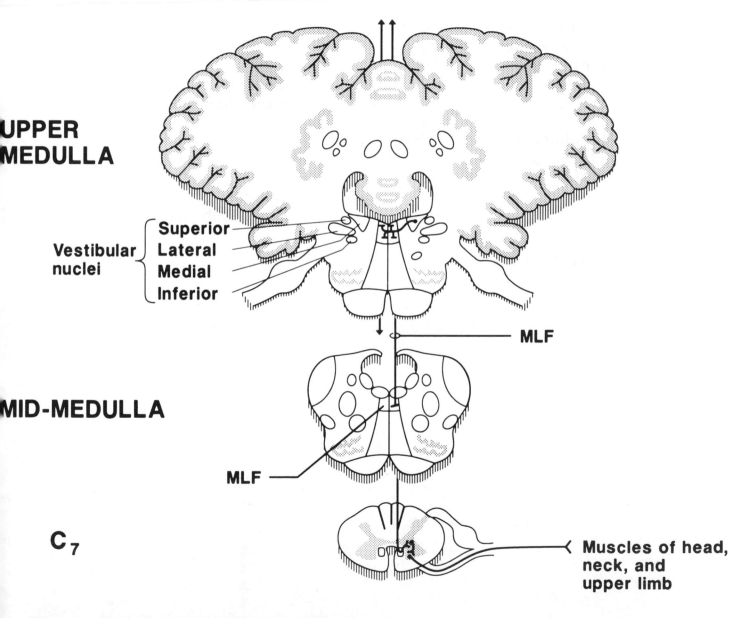

UPPER MEDULLA

Vestibular nuclei {
Superior
Lateral
Medial
Inferior

MLF

MID-MEDULLA

MLF

C₇

Muscles of head, neck, and upper limb

Figure 30 **Medial longitudinal fasciculus (MLF)**

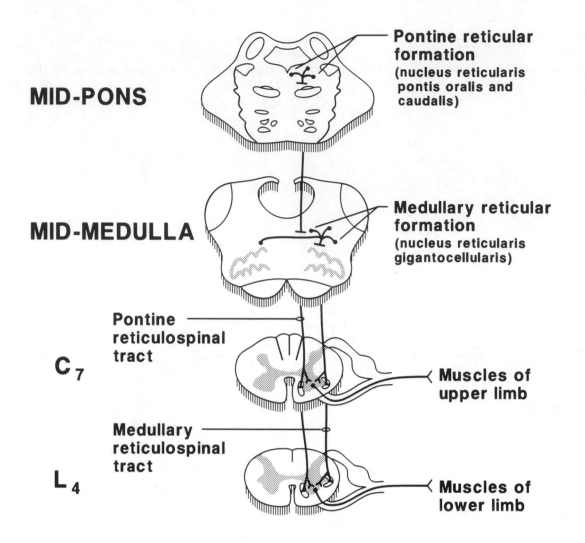

MID-PONS

Pontine reticular formation
(nucleus reticularis pontis oralis and caudalis)

MID-MEDULLA

Medullary reticular formation
(nucleus reticularis gigantocellularis)

Pontine reticulospinal tract

C 7

Muscles of upper limb

Medullary reticulospinal tract

L 4

Muscles of lower limb

Figure 31   Reticulospinal tracts

Spinal (Paleocerebellar) Connections
(Figures 29, 31–35)

1. Input
   a. Sensory information (particularly unconscious proprioception from neuromuscular and neurotendinous spindles) carried in the *anterior* and *posterior spinocerebellar tracts* and the *cuneocerebellar tract* reaches the cerebellum via the following pathways (Figure 32)
   b. Anterior spinocerebellar tract
      (1) Receptors
         (a) Neurotendinous spindles (Golgi)
      (2) Peripheral processes of pseudounipolar cell bodies (dendrites)
         (a) Heavily myelinated fibers (Aα, Ib) in peripheral nerves
         (b) Converge on the spinal nerves
         (c) Enter the dorsal roots of the lumbar and sacral spinal nerves
      (3) Cell bodies of the first-order neurons
         (a) Large pseudounipolar cell bodies in the lumbar and sacral spinal ganglia
      (4) Central processes of the pseudounipolar cell bodies (axons)
         (a) Enter the spinal cord through the medial division of the dorsal root
      (5) First synapse
         (a) Posterior horn of the lumbar and sacral segments of the spinal cord
      (6) Course of axons of the second-order neurons
         (a) Cross to the contralateral side of the cord through the white commissure
         (b) Enter the *anterior spinocerebellar tract* in the anterior part of the lateral funiculus
         (c) Ascend in the cord to the medulla
         (d) Ascend through the lateral field of the brain stem to upper pontine levels, enter the cerebellum along the superior cerebellar peduncle, and recross within the cerebellum to the original ipsilateral side of the cerebellum
         (e) End in the vermis of the cerebellum
   c. Posterior spinocerebellar tract
      (1) Receptors
         (a) Neuromuscular spindles (anulospiral and flower-spray endings)
         (b) Neurotendinous spindles (Golgi)
      (2) Peripheral processes of pseudounipolar cell bodies (dendrites)
         (a) Heavily myelinated fibers (Aα, Ia and Ib) in peripheral nerves
         (b) Converge on the spinal nerves
         (c) Enter the dorsal roots of the spinal nerves
      (3) Cell bodies of the first-order neurons
         (a) Large pseudounipolar cell bodies in the spinal ganglia
      (4) Central processes of the pseudounipolar cell bodies (axons)
         (a) Enter the spinal cord through the medial division of the dorsal root
         (b) Fibers from spinal ganglia below the third lumbar segment of the cord pass into the ipsilateral fasciculus gracilis and ascend to the third lumbar segment of the cord (or slightly above)
         (c) Fibers from spinal ganglia above the first thoracic segment of the cord pass into the ipsilateral fasciculus cuneatus and ascend to the medulla
      (5) First synapse
         (a) Thoracic nucleus (nucl. dorsalis, Clarke's nucl.) of the spinal cord (from T_1 to L_3) — fibers from spinal ganglia below the first thoracic level of the cord synapse in the thoracic nucleus
         (b) Accessory cuneate nucleus of the medulla — fibers from spinal ganglia above the first thoracic level of the cord synapse in this nucleus
      (6) Course of axons of the second-order neurons
         (a) From the thoracic nucleus
            i. Axons swing laterally to enter the *posterior spinocerebellar tract* in the posterior part of the ipsilateral lateral funiculus
            ii. Ascend in the cord to the medulla
            iii. In the medulla, the tract gradually passes posteriorly, peripheral to the spinal tract of the trigeminal nerve, to enter the *inferior cerebellar peduncle*
            iv. Enter the ipsilateral side of the cerebellum through the inferior cerebellar peduncle
            v. End in the vermis of the cerebellum
         (b) From the accessory cuneate nucleus
            i. Axons swing laterally as the *cuneocerebellar tract* and enter the *inferior cerebellar peduncle*
            ii. Enter the ipsilateral side of the cerebellum through the inferior cerebellar peduncle
            iii. End in the paravermal (intermediate) hemisphere of the cerebellum

13523

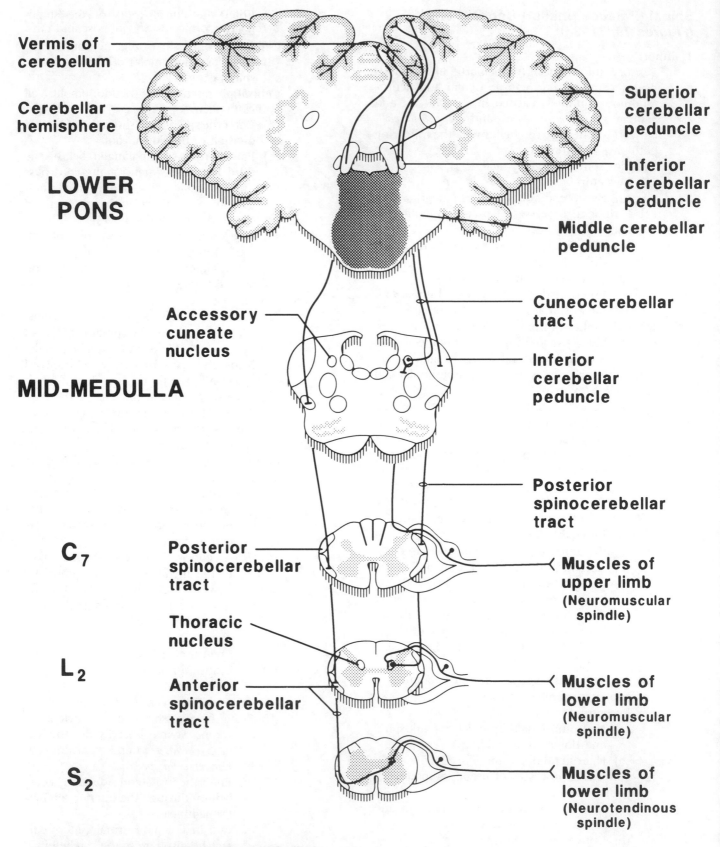

LOWER PONS

Vermis of cerebellum

Cerebellar hemisphere

Superior cerebellar peduncle

Inferior cerebellar peduncle

Middle cerebellar peduncle

Cuneocerebellar tract

Accessory cuneate nucleus

MID-MEDULLA

Inferior cerebellar peduncle

Posterior spinocerebellar tract

C₇

Posterior spinocerebellar tract

Muscles of upper limb (Neuromuscular spindle)

Thoracic nucleus

L₂

Anterior spinocerebellar tract

Muscles of lower limb (Neuromuscular spindle)

S₂

Muscles of lower limb (Neurotendinous spindle)

Figure 32 Spinocerebellar (paleocerebellar) connections: input

d. Within the cerebellum, these fibers end as the mossy fibers of the *paleocerebellum* [vermis and paravermal (intermediate) hemisphere]

e. The mossy fibers synapse with granule cells, which in turn synapse with Purkinje cells

2. Output

a. The Purkinje cells of the vermis project to the fastigial nucleus

   (1) The cells of the fastigial nucleus send their axons out of the cerebellum mainly through the *inferior cerebellar peduncle*

   (2) These fibers end in the brain stem reticular formation and the vestibular nuclei and thereby influence lower motor neurons by way of the reticulospinal and vestibulospinal tracts (Figures 29 and 31)

b. The Purkinje cells of the paravermal (intermediate) hemisphere project to the globose and emboliform nuclei

   (1) The cells of the globose and emboliform nuclei send their axons out of the cerebellum through the *superior cerebellar peduncle*

   (2) These fibers cross to the contralateral side of the brain stem in the *decussation of the superior cerebellar peduncle* and end in the red nucleus. They influence lower motor neurons by way of the *rubrospinal tract* (Figure 35)

3. Function

a. Regulation of muscle tone

b. Regulation of the execution and coordination of limb movements

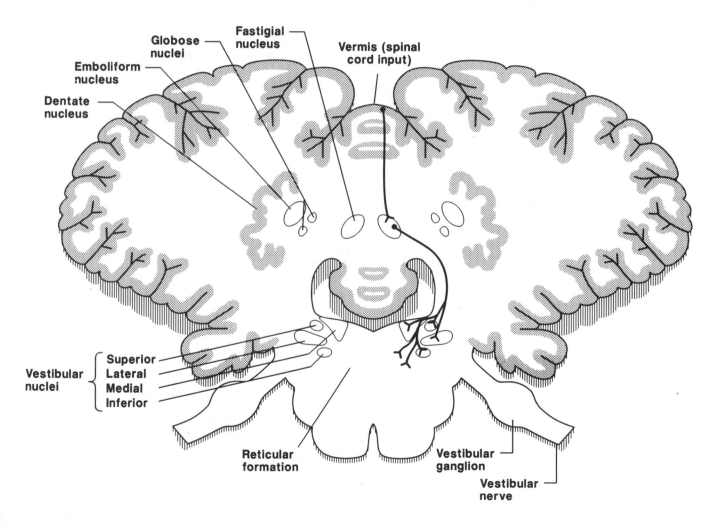

Figure 33 Spinocerebellar (paleocerebellar) connections: output I

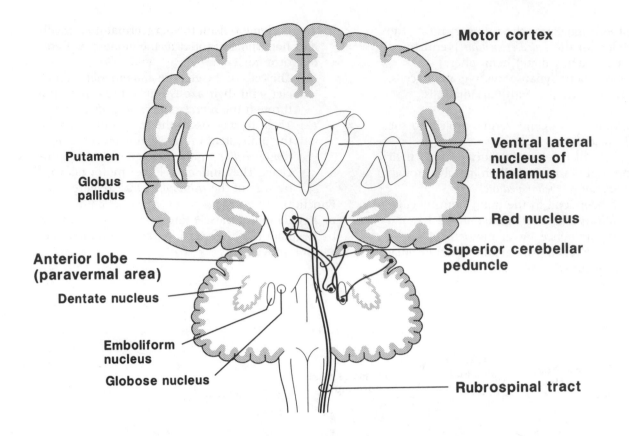

Figure 34 **Spinocerebellar (paleocerebellar) connections: output II**

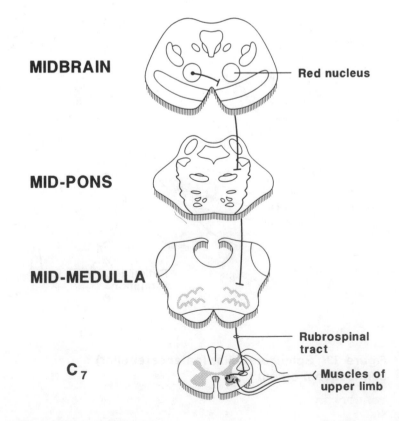

Figure 35 **Rubrospinal tract**

Cortical (Neocerebellar) Connections (Figure 36)

1. Input
   a. Information from the cerebral cortex (especially concerning somatic motor functioning) descends through the internal capsule and midbrain in the *corticopontine tracts* (and perhaps also as collaterals from the corticospinal and corticonuclear tracts)
   b. In the pons, these tracts synapse with *pontine nuclei* in the ipsilateral side of the anterior (basilar) part of the pons
   c. The axons of these cells form the pontocerebellar fibers, which cross to the contralateral side of the pons and enter the *middle cerebellar peduncle*
   d. These fibers enter the cerebellum through the middle cerebellar peduncle and end as the mossy fibers of the *neocerebellum* (or lateral hemisphere)
   e. The mossy fibers synapse with granule cells, which in turn synapse with Purkinje cells
2. Output
   a. The Purkinje cells of the neocerebellum project to the dentate nucleus of the cerebellum
   b. The cells of the dentate nucleus send their axons into the *dentatorubrothalamic tract*, which passes out of the cerebellum through the *superior cerebellar peduncle*
   c. The dentatorubrothalamic tract crosses to the contralateral side of the brain stem in the decussation of the superior cerebellar peduncle at the inferior collicular level of the midbrain
   d. Some of the fibers of the tract synapse with cells in the red nucleus, but most pass around the red nucleus without synapsing
   e. The tract, including fibers from the red nucleus, continues to ascend and ends in the *ventral lateral nucleus of the thalamus*
   f. Fibers from the ventral lateral nucleus of the thalamus project to the (original ipsilateral) motor and premotor cortices (areas 4 and 6), thereby completing an important feedback loop for the control of motor activity
3. Function
   a. Regulation of the planning, initiation, timing, and coordination of discrete movements of the limbs, eyes, and vocal apparatus

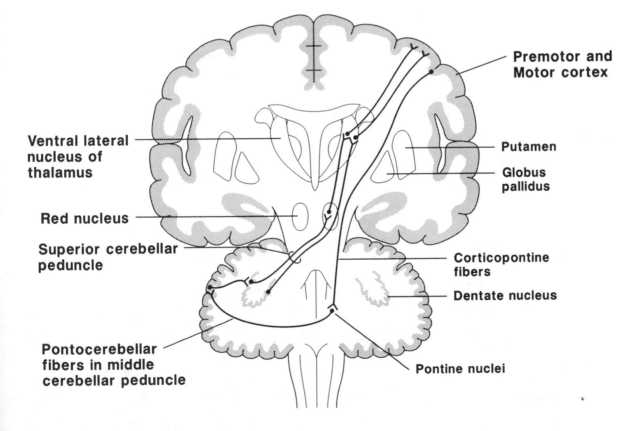

Figure 36   Corticocerebellar (neocerebellar) connections

Olivocerebellar Connections
(Figure 37)

1. Input to the inferior olivary nucleus
   a. Spinal cord via the spino-olivary tract
   b. Central tegmental tract — with fibers, directly or indirectly, from the red nucleus, central gray substance of the midbrain, and cerebral cortex
2. Output from the inferior olivary nucleus
   a. Olivocerebellar fibers cross the median plane, enter the cerebellum through the *inferior cerebellar peduncle,* and project to all parts of the cerebellar cortex as climbing fibers.
   b. The climbing fibers synapse with Purkinje cells
3. Output from the cerebellum
   a. The Purkinje cells project to the deep cerebellar nuclei (predominantly the dentate nucleus)
   b. The cells of the dentate nucleus send their axons out of the cerebellum through the *superior cerebellar peduncle*
   c. At the inferior collicular level of the midbrain, the superior cerebellar peduncle decussates to the opposite side
   d. The fibers synapse with cells in the red nucleus, which send their axons into the central tegmental tract
   e. The central tegmental tract descends through the brain stem to the ipsilateral inferior olivary nucleus, thereby completing another feedback loop in the cerebellar system
4. Function
   a. These connections may be involved in aspects of learning motor tasks

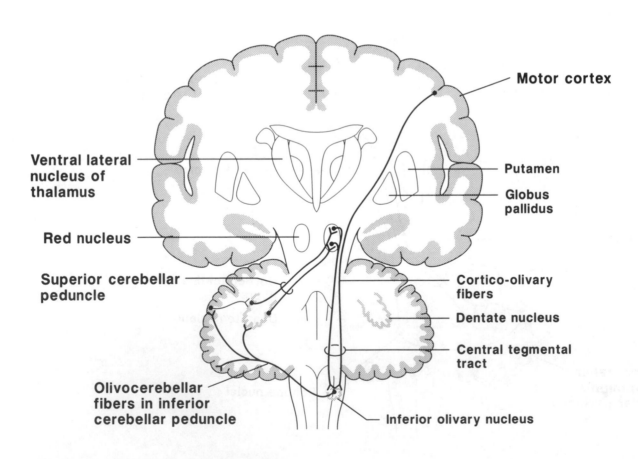

Motor cortex

Ventral lateral nucleus of thalamus

Putamen

Globus pallidus

Red nucleus

Superior cerebellar peduncle

Cortico-olivary fibers

Dentate nucleus

Central tegmental tract

Olivocerebellar fibers in inferior cerebellar peduncle

Inferior olivary nucleus

Figure 37 **Olivocerebellar connections**

CONNECTIONS OF THE BASAL NUCLEI

The term *basal nuclei* (often still erroneously referred to as "basal ganglia") refers to a group of subcortical masses of gray matter located deep in the cerebral hemispheres. Included in this group of nuclei are the caudate nucleus, putamen, globus pallidus, claustrum, and amygdaloid body. The claustrum is of obscure significance and the amygdaloid body is a functional component of the limbic and olfactory systems. Neither will be considered further in this discussion. However, the subthalamic nucleus and the substantia nigra, although not structurally included in the basal nuclei, are closely related to them in a functional sense. The terminology concerning the basal nuclei can be confusing. The following comparative terms are helpful in sorting through this confusion:

(1) Striatum (neostriatum) = caudate nucleus and putamen

(2) Pallidum (paleostriatum) = globus pallidus
(3) Lentiform nucleus = putamen and globus pallidus

By the number and complexity of the interconnections within the basal nuclei, it is assumed that they function as a modulating and integrating center concerning motor activity. They receive impressive input from the cerebral cortex. This information is projected to the *ventral lateral* and *ventral anterior nuclei of the thalamus* and directed toward the motor areas of the cerebral cortex. Therefore, it appears that the basal nuclei exert most of their influence on and through the cerebral cortex rather than directly on the brain stem nuclei that give rise to descending motor pathways. In this sense they are functionally similar to the neocerebellum as opposed to the older parts of the cerebellum, which have more direct connections with brain stem nuclei such as the reticular formation, red nucleus, and vestibular nuclei. See Figure 38 for a schematic representation of the connections of the basal nuclei and the main neurotransmitters involved in those connections.

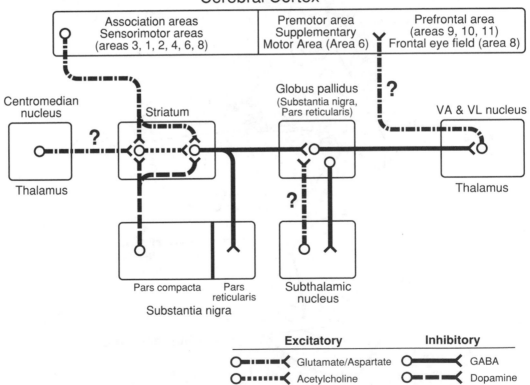

Figure 38 Schematic diagram of the connections of the basal nuclei

The basal nuclei are important in complex, stereotyped, supporting muscular activities such as postural adjustments, balance, locomotion, and associated movements (e.g., arm swinging during walking, "righting movements," gestures). They seem to mediate their functions via feedback loops or circuits that project back up to the frontal cortex (especially the supplementary motor area) for the planning, initiation, and execution of movements. In this way certain movements and behaviors may be "selected" and other unwanted movements may be "suppressed." These feedback circuits are outlined below as a series of afferent (input) and efferent (output) connections of the striatum and pallidum.

Striatal (Caudate Nucleus and Putamen) Connections
(Figures 39 and 40)

1. Input
   a. Corticostriate fibers
      (1) A widespread projection from all parts of the cortex, but especially from motor (frontal) and sensory (parietal) areas
      (2) Fibers enter the caudate and putamen via the internal and external capsules
      (3) These inputs are excitatory and utilize glutamate and/or aspartate as their neurotransmitter

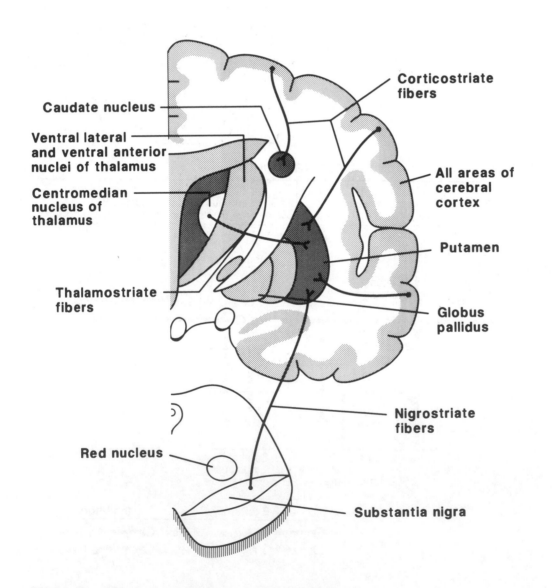

Figure 39 **Afferent connections of the striatum (caudate and putamen)**

b. Nigrostriate fibers
   (1) A dopaminergic pathway from the substantia nigra (pars compacta), which is ipsilateral and inhibitory
   (2) Many interneurons within the striatum are cholinergic (excitatory) and form a counterbalanced system with the dopaminergic nigrostriatal system
c. Thalamostriate fibers
   (1) Fibers from the centromedian nucleus and other intralaminar nuclei of the thalamus
   (2) An excitatory pathway, probably utilizing glutamate

2. Output
   a. Striopallidal fibers — to the globus pallidus (major pathway), utilizing γ-aminobutyric acid (GABA) as an inhibitory neurotransmitter
   b. Strionigral fibers — an inhibitory feedback loop with the substantia nigra (pars reticularis) using GABA

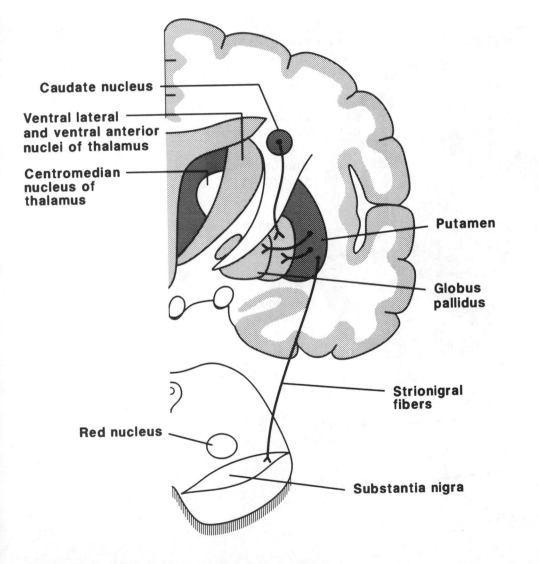

Caudate nucleus

Ventral lateral and ventral anterior nuclei of thalamus

Centromedian nucleus of thalamus

Putamen

Globus pallidus

Strionigral fibers

Red nucleus

Substantia nigra

Figure 40 **Efferent connections of the striatum (caudate and putamen)**

Pallidal (Globus Pallidus) Connections (Figures 41 and 42)

1. Input
   a. Striopallidal fibers — from the caudate and putamen (the largest afferent input), an inhibitory pathway utilizing GABA
   b. Subthalamopallidal fibers — an ipsilateral, probably excitatory pathway (glutamate) from the subthalamic nucleus to the globus pallidus through the *subthalamic fasciculus*
2. Output
   a. Pallidothalamic fibers

(1) Fibers from the globus pallidus enter the *lenticular fasciculus* and *ansa lenticularis* (which join to form the *thalamic fasciculus*) and project to the *ventral lateral* and *ventral anterior nuclei of the thalamus*

(2) These nuclei project back up to the *supplementary motor area,* (premotor area), frontal eye field (area 8), and prefrontal area of the cerebral cortex, thereby bringing these areas under the regulatory influence of the basal nuclei. The pallidothalamic fibers are inhibitory and GABAergic, whereas the thalamocortical projections are excitatory and may

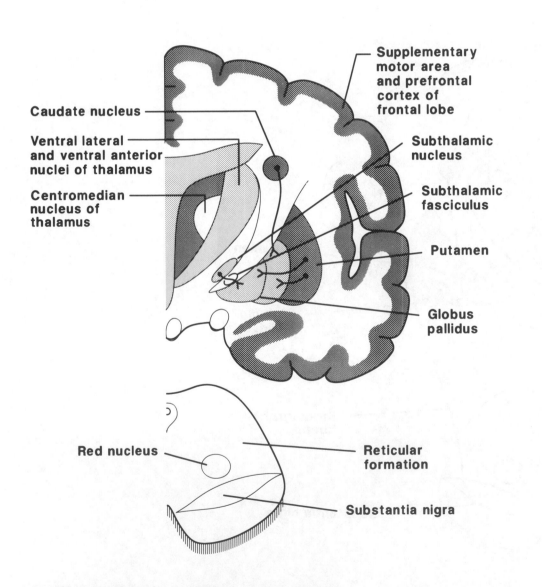

Figure 41   Afferent connections of the pallidum (globus pallidus)

utilize glutamate as their neurotransmitter.

b. Pallidosubthalamic fibers — an inhibitory feed-back loop to the subthalamic nucleus via the subthalamic fasciculus using GABA

c. Efferent fibers project to the midbrain reticular formation, which in turn projects to other nuclei that give rise to descending motor pathways (rubrospinal, reticulospinal, vestibulospinal tracts).

Figures 43 and 44 are schematic representations of the basic connections and pathways involved in the control of voluntary motor activity and serve as a summary of many of the preceding sections.

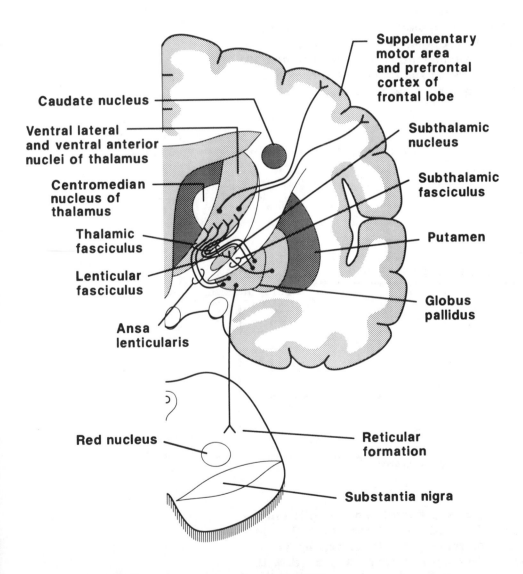

Figure 42 **Efferent connections of the pallidum (globus pallidus)**

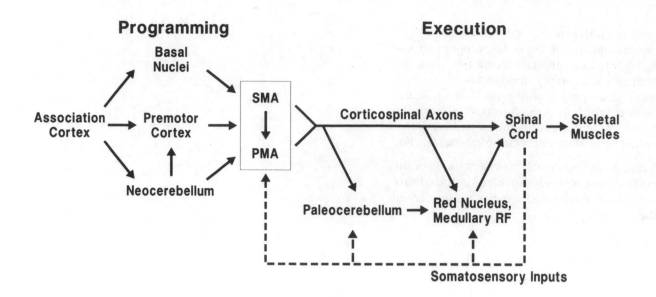

Figure 43 Control of voluntary motor activity: afferent and efferent connections of the primary (PMA) and supplementary (SMA) motor areas. (Adapted from: Humphrey, D.R. Corticospinal systems and their control by premotor cortex, basal ganglia, and cerebellum. Chapter 19 in *Neurobiology*, assoc. ed. W.D. Willis. In *The Clinical Neurosciences*, ed. R.N. Rosenberg. Churchill Livingstone, New York, 1983.)

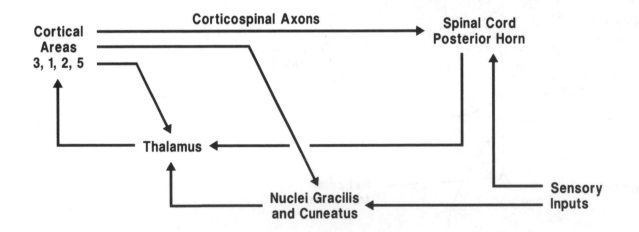

Figure 44 Control of voluntary motor activity: afferent and efferent connections of the parietal lobe. (Adapted from: Humphrey, D.R. Corticospinal systems and their control by premotor cortex, basal ganglia, and cerebellum. Chapter 19 in *Neurobiology*, Assoc. ed. W.D. Willis. In *The Clinical Neurosciences*, ed. R.N. Rosenberg. Churchill Livingstone, New York, 1983.)

Part Three

Blood Vessels of the Brain and Spinal Cord

Blood Vessels of the Brain

ARTERIAL SUPPLY TO THE BRAIN

The brain is supplied by two pairs of arteries, the *internal carotid arteries* (the "anterior circulation") and the *vertebral arteries* (the "posterior circulation"). These arteries arise from the three main arterial branches of the aortic arch: the *brachiocephalic trunk*, which divides into the right subclavian artery and the right common carotid artery, the *left common carotid artery*, and the *left subclavian artery* (Figure 45).

Internal Carotid Artery (the "Anterior Circulation")

1. Origin
   a. The internal carotid artery arises from the bifurcation of the common carotid artery at the upper border of the thyroid cartilage of the larynx. It can be divided into four named segments: cervical, petrous, cavernous, and cerebral (supraclinoid) (Figures 45–47).
2. Course
   a. The *cervical segment* ascends in the neck posterior and medial to the external carotid artery and has no branches. At the base of the skull it enters the carotid canal of the petrous part of the temporal bone.
   b. The *petrous segment* ascends a short distance, then turns anteromedially, and finally exits the carotid canal near the apex of the petrous bone to cross over the foramen lacerum and enter the cavernous sinus. It has two small branches of little significance.
   c. The *cavernous segment* passes anteriorly within the cavernous sinus in close relation to cranial nerves III, IV, V, and VI. It then passes superomedially and posteriorly to pierce the dura mater just medial to the anterior clinoid process. It has several small branches to the sinus itself, the pituitary gland, the trigeminal ganglion, and adjacent meninges. The *ophthalmic artery* arises at the point where the internal carotid pierces the dura.

It passes through the optic canal into the orbit inferolateral to the optic nerve (II).
   d. The *cerebral (supraclinoid) segment* ascends posteriorly, and passes between the oculomotor and optic nerves to reach the medial end of the lateral sulcus, where it ends by dividing into its terminal branches, the *anterior* and *middle cerebral arteries* (Figures 46, 48, 56, and 57). The cavernous and supraclinoid parts of the internal carotid artery are known as the *carotid siphon*. Aside from small branches to adjacent structures (e.g., optic chiasma, pituitary gland), this segment of the internal carotid artery gives off two important branches, the *posterior communicating artery* and the *anterior choroidal artery*.
      (1) The *posterior communicating artery* courses posteriorly and medially beneath the optic tract to join the posterior cerebral artery. It supplies small branches to the optic tract, hypothalamus, thalamus, and cerebral peduncles.
      (2) The *anterior choroidal artery* arises just distal to the posterior communicating artery and follows the optic tract and cerebral peduncle as far as the lateral geniculate body, where it enters the choroid plexus of the inferior horn of the lateral ventricle. In its course it passes just medial to the uncus. It supplies branches to the optic tract, the genu, posterior limb, and retrolentiform parts of the internal capsule, the globus pallidus, adjacent parts of the temporal lobe, midbrain, and thalamus.
3. Branches of the anterior and middle cerebral arteries
   a. The *anterior cerebral artery* passes anteriorly and medially above the optic nerve to enter the longitudinal cerebral fissure. There it is joined with the opposite anterior cerebral artery by the short *anterior communicating artery*. The artery then swings upward and posteriorly over the rostrum and genu of the corpus callosum and continues posteriorly on the superior aspect of the corpus callosum as far as the parieto-occipital sulcus (Figures 46–48, 56, and 57).

Figure 45A **The origin and course of the internal carotid and vertebral arteries**

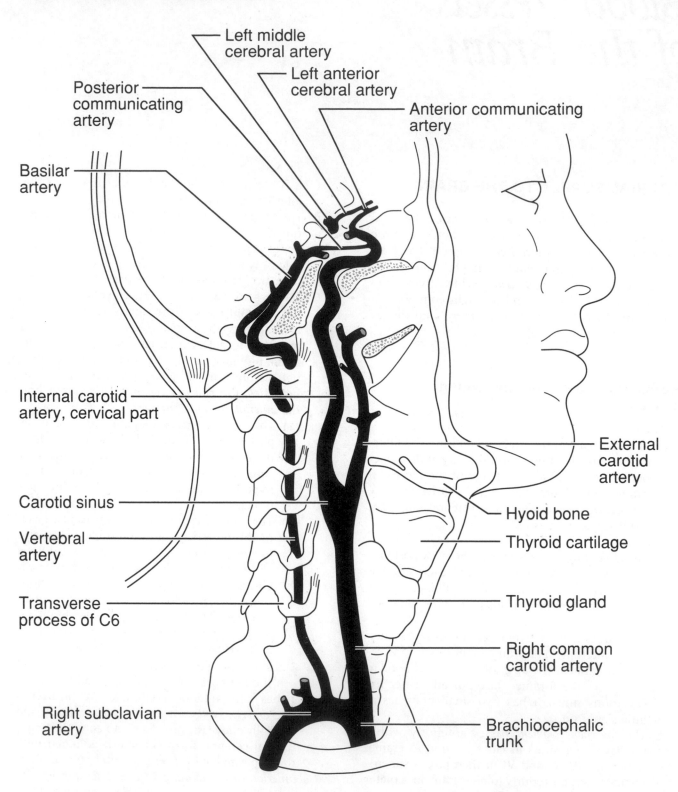

Left middle cerebral artery

Left anterior cerebral artery

Posterior communicating artery

Anterior communicating artery

Basilar artery

Internal carotid artery, cervical part

External carotid artery

Carotid sinus

Hyoid bone

Vertebral artery

Thyroid cartilage

Transverse process of C6

Thyroid gland

Right common carotid artery

Right subclavian artery

Brachiocephalic trunk

Figure 45B   Subtraction angiogram of the right carotid arterial system, lateral view

A. Common carotid artery
B. Internal carotid artery, cervical part
C. External carotid artery
D. Internal carotid artery, cavernous part
E. Anterior cerebral artery
F. Branches of middle cerebral artery

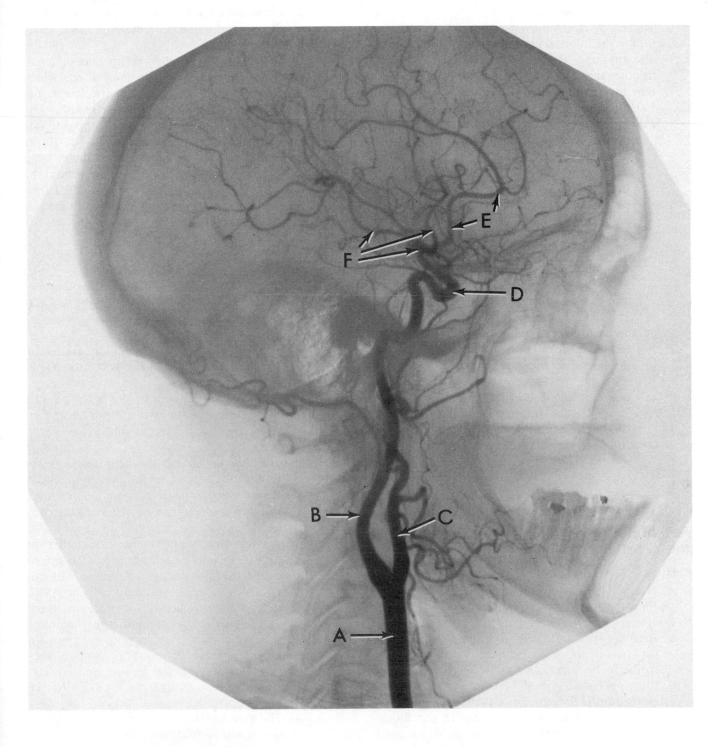

(1) The *cortical branches* of the anterior cerebral artery ramify on the medial aspect of the frontal and parietal lobes and over onto the superior gyri of the lateral surface of the hemisphere (Figures 46 and 47).

(2) The *central branches* of the anterior cerebral artery supply the anterior hypothalamus, the septal region, the antero-inferior parts of the basal nuclei, and the anterior limb of the internal capsule.

b. The *middle cerebral artery* is the direct continuation of the internal carotid artery. It passes laterally inferior to the anterior perforated substance to enter the lateral sulcus, where it divides into two to four branches (Figures 46–48, 56, and 57).

(1) These *cortical branches* course upward and posteriorly over the insula, execute a hairpin turn at its upper border, descend over the inner surface of the operculum, and exit from the lateral sulcus to spread superiorly over the lateral aspect of the frontal, parietal, and occipital lobes and inferiorly over the lateral aspect of the temporal lobe. The terminal branches of the middle cerebral artery anastomose with those of the anterior and posterior cerebral arteries (Figures 46 and 47).

(2) The *central branches* of the middle cerebral artery (anterolateral or lenticulostriate arteries) arise from the superior surface of the horizontal segment of the artery, pass superiorly and posteriorly to penetrate the anterior perforated substance, and supply the lateral part of the globus pallidus, putamen, caudate, superior part of the internal capsule, and corona radiata (Figure 46).

Vertebral Artery (the "Posterior Circulation")

1. Origin
   a. The vertebral artery arises as the first branch of the subclavian artery (Figure 45).
2. Course
   a. It passes superomedially to enter the transverse foramen of the sixth cervical vertebra, ascends through the succeeding transverse foramina of the upper six cervical vertebrae, winds posteriorly around the superior articular process of the atlas, and pierces the atlantooccipital membrane and dura mater to enter the posterior fossa through the foramen magnum (Figure 45).

b. Intracranially, the vertebral artery ascends anteriorly and medially around the medulla to reach the midline at the pontomedullary junction, where it joins the vertebral artery from the other side to form the *basilar artery* (Figures 45, 48, 49, 56, and 57).

3. Branches
   a. In the neck, the vertebral artery gives off multiple *muscular* and *spinal branches*. The spinal branches pass through the intervertebral foramina to supply the cervical spinal cord, meninges, and vertebrae.
   b. Intracranially, the vertebral artery gives off a meningeal branch; the *posterior spinal artery*, which supplies the posterior aspect of the lower medulla and spinal cord; the *anterior spinal artery*, which unites with its fellow of the opposite side and supplies the anteromedial aspect of the lower medulla and spinal cord; and the *posterior inferior cerebellar artery*, which winds around the lateral aspect of the medulla to supply the lateral medulla and the posterior aspect of the inferior surface of the cerebellum (Figures 48, 49, 56, and 57).

4. Basilar artery
   a. Origin
      (1) The *basilar artery* originates at the pontomedullary junction by the union of the two vertebral arteries.
   b. Course
      (1) It passes superiorly in a shallow groove on the anterior surface of the pons (the *basilar sulcus*).
      (2) It ends at the superior border of the pons by bifurcating into the two *posterior cerebral arteries* (Figures 48, 49, 56, and 57).
   c. Branches
      (1) The *anterior inferior cerebellar artery* wraps around the anterolateral aspect of the lower pons to supply the lateral pons and the anterior aspect of the inferior surface of the cerebellum.
      (2) The *labyrinthine artery* arises from either the basilar or anterior inferior cerebellar artery, enters the internal acoustic canal with the facial (VII) and vestibulocochlear (VIII) nerves, and supplies the inner ear structures.
      (3) The *pontine arteries* are numerous small vessels, which penetrate the pons to supply the medial (paramedian group), anterolateral (short circumferential group), and posterolateral (long circumferential group) aspects of the pons.
      (4) The *superior cerebellar artery* arises just proximal to the termination of the basilar artery, and passes laterally just inferior to the oculo-

motor nerve (III) to wind around the pons–midbrain junction to supply the lateral and posterior aspects of the upper pons and midbrain and the superior surface of the cerebellum.

(5) The *posterior cerebral artery* arises at the superior border of the pons by the terminal bifurcation of the basilar artery. It passes laterally parallel to the superior cerebellar artery and is separated from it by the oculomotor nerve and the tentorium cerebelli. Receiving the posterior communicating artery, it winds around the cerebral peduncle to supply the midbrain, the hypothalamus, the thalamus, the geniculate bodies, and the choroid plexus of the third and lateral ventricles via *central* or *penetrating branches*. *Cortical branches* of the artery ramify on the inferior and medial aspects of the temporal and occipital lobes, as well as slightly over onto the lateral surface of the hemisphere to anastomose with terminal branches of the middle cerebral artery (Figures 47–49, 56, and 57).

The Cerebral Arterial Circle

The *cerebral arterial circle* (Willis) is an anastomotic communication between the anterior (carotid) and posterior (vertebrobasilar) circulations, as well as between the left and right sides of the cerebral circulation. It is located at the base of the brain encircling the optic chiasma, tuber cinereum, and interpeduncular fossa. It is formed by the *anterior* and *posterior communicating arteries* and the proximal portions of the *anterior, middle,* and *posterior cerebral arteries*. It serves to equalize the blood flow to various parts of the brain in the event of an occlusion of one or more of the major arteries contributing to the circle. Unfortunately, often one of the three "communicating" arteries of the circle is either absent or hypoplastic, thereby causing this potential anastomosis to functionally fail (Figures 48, 56, and 57).

A. Internal carotid artery, cervical part
B. Internal carotid artery, petrous part
C. Internal carotid artery, cavernous part
D. Internal carotid artery, cerebral (supraclinoid) part
E. Right anterior cerebral artery
F. Anterior communicating artery
G. Left anterior cerebral artery (cross-filled from right anterior cerebral artery through the anterior communicating artery)
H. Right and left pericallosal branches of anterior cerebral arteries

I. Cortical branches of anterior cerebral arteries
J. Anterior choroidal artery
K. Middle cerebral artery
L. Anterolateral central (lenticulostriate) branches of middle cerebral artery
M. Cortical branches of middle cerebral artery

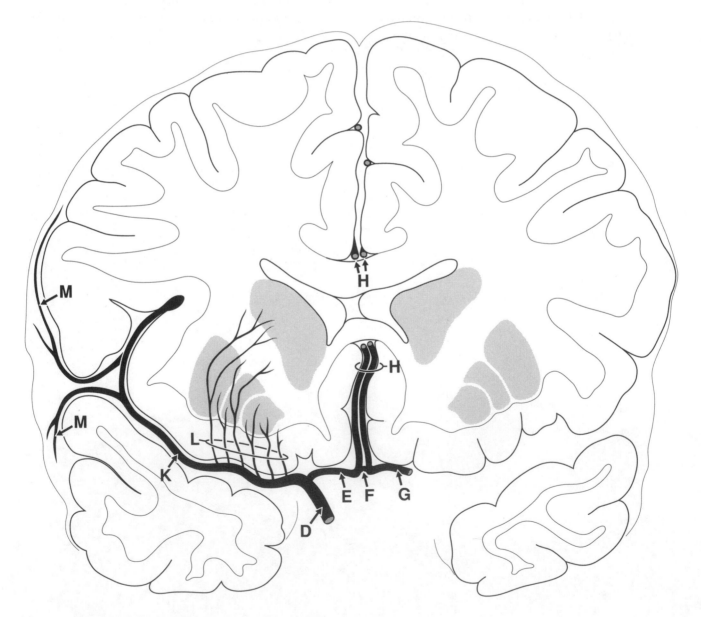

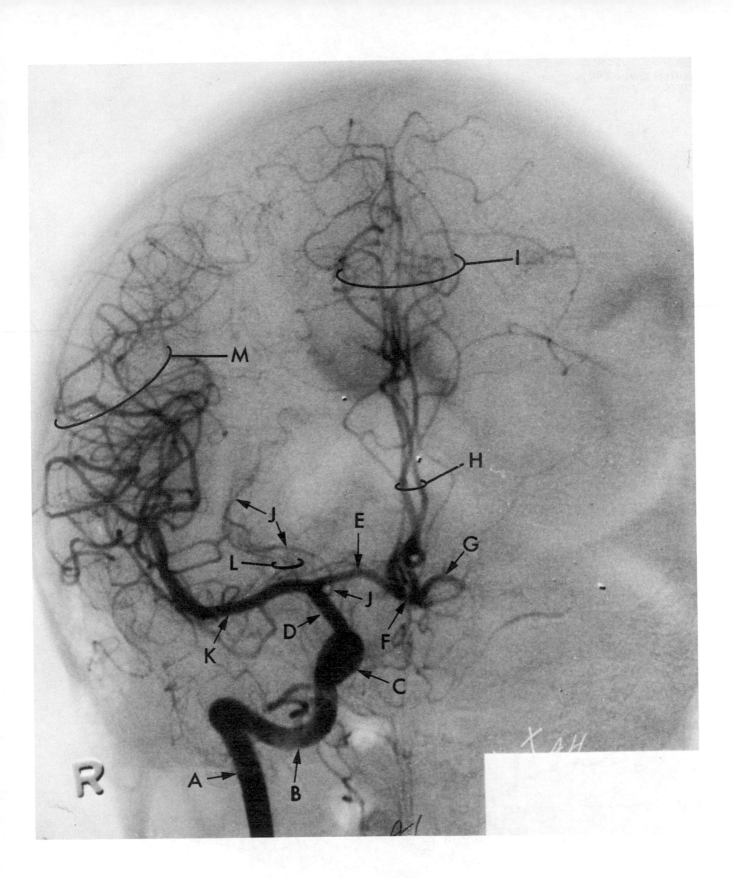

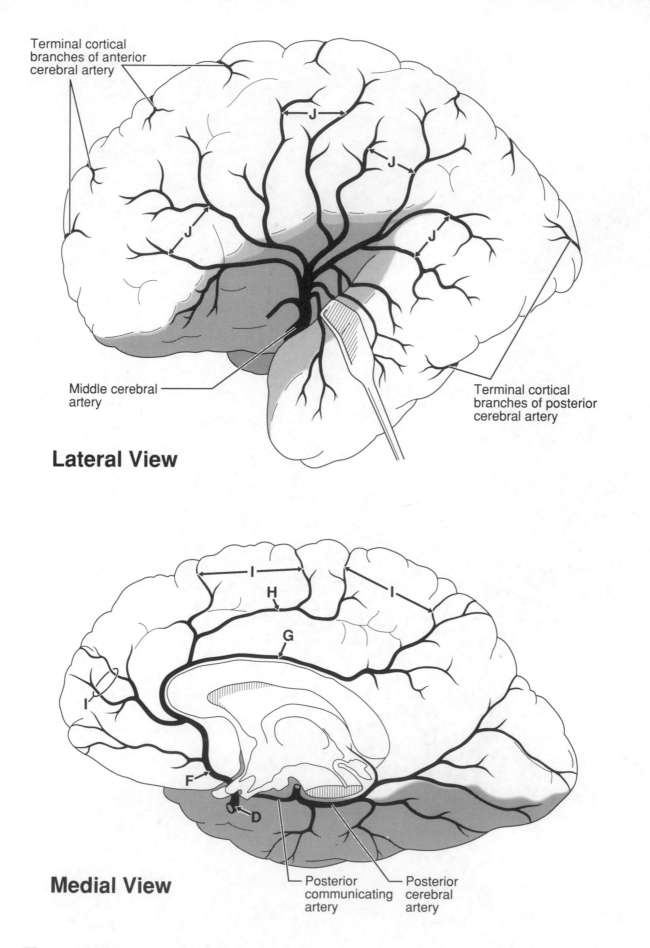

Terminal cortical
branches of anterior
cerebral artery

J

J

J

J

Middle cerebral
artery

Terminal cortical
branches of posterior
cerebral artery

Lateral View

I

H

I

G

I

F

D

Posterior
communicating
artery

Posterior
cerebral
artery

Medial View

Figure 47 **Subtraction angiogram of the left
internal carotid artery, lateral view**

A. Internal carotid artery, cervical part
B. Internal carotid artery, petrous part
C. Internal carotid artery, cavernous part
D. Internal carotid artery, cerebral (supraclinoid) part
E. Ophthalmic artery
F. Right and left anterior cerebral arteries (right side cross-filled from the left)

G. Pericallosal branch of anterior cerebral artery
H. Left and right callosomarginal branches of anterior cerebral arteries
I. Cortical branches of anterior cerebral artery
J. Cortical branches of middle cerebral artery

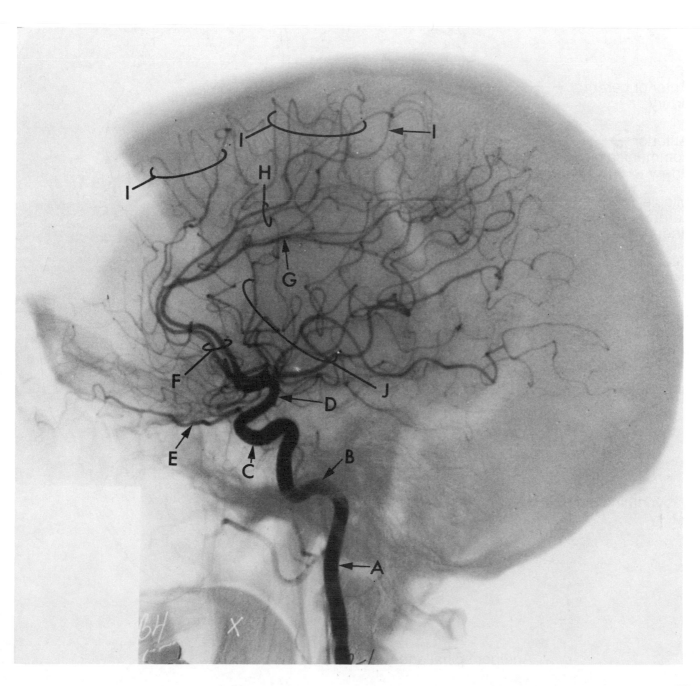

Figure 48 **Subtraction angiogram of the vertebrobasilar arterial system, posterior–anterior view**

A. Vertebral arteries
B. Posterior inferior cerebellar artery
C. Anterior inferior cerebellar artery
D. Basilar artery
E. Superior cerebellar artery
F. Posterior cerebral arteries
G. Cortical branches of posterior cerebral arteries

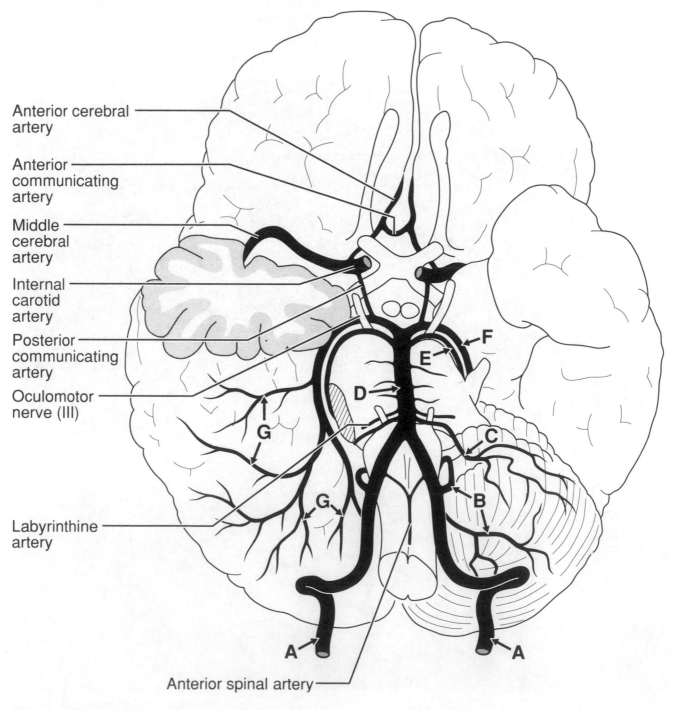

Anterior cerebral artery

Anterior communicating artery

Middle cerebral artery

Internal carotid artery

Posterior communicating artery

Oculomotor nerve (III)

Labyrinthine artery

Anterior spinal artery

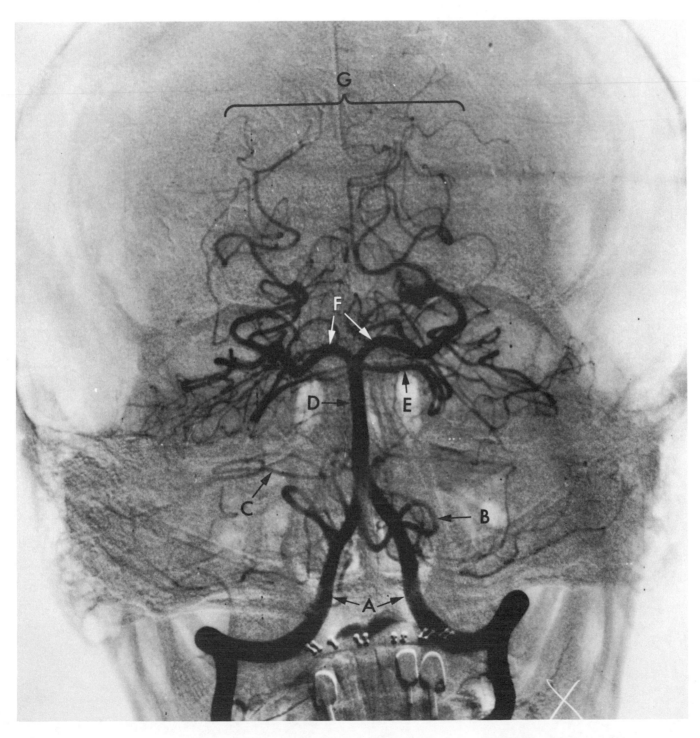

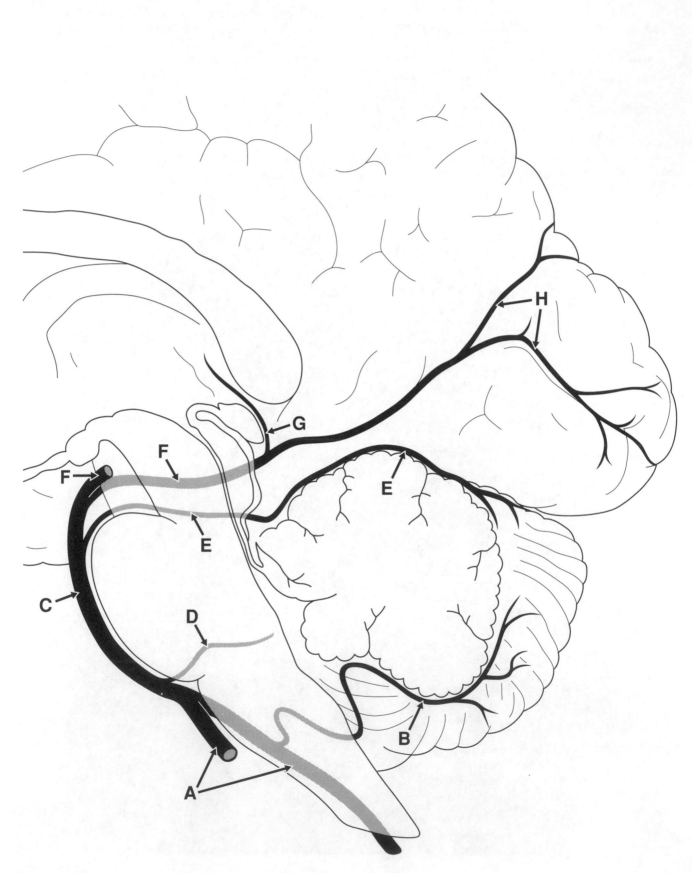

Figure 49 Subtraction angiogram of the
vertebrobasilar arterial system, left lateral view

A. Vertebral arteries
B. Right and left posterior inferior cerebellar
   arteries
C. Basilar artery
D. Anterior inferior cerebellar artery
E. Superior cerebellar arteries
F. Posterior cerebral arteries

G. Posterolateral central (thalamogeniculate)
   branches of posterior cerebral arteries
   (including posterior choroidal arteries)
H. Cortical branches of posterior cerebral arteries
I. Posteromedial central (thalamoperforating)
   branches of posterior cerebral arteries

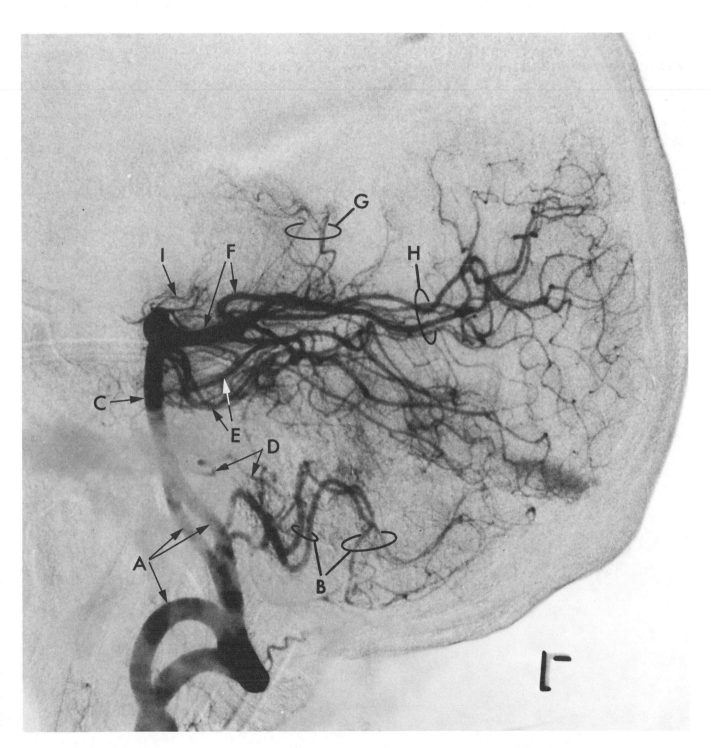

VENOUS RETURN FROM THE BRAIN

The veins of the brain are thin walled and have no valves. They do not run with the cerebral arteries, but course independently, and are usually divided into superficial and deep groups. These veins eventually empty, either directly or indirectly, into a system of intercommunicating endothelium-lined channels known as the *sinuses of the dura mater*. The dural venous sinuses ultimately empty into the two *internal jugular veins*, which receive almost the entire venous drainage from the brain.

Venous Sinuses of the Dura Mater

The dural venous sinuses are located either between the periosteal and meningeal layers of the dura mater or within foldings of the meningeal layer. The sinuses are grouped into a posterosuperior group of midline sinuses and their continuations (numbers one to six below) and an anteroinferior group of paired sinuses related to the cavernous sinuses (numbers seven to eleven below) (Figures 50–52).

1. The *superior sagittal sinus* begins at the foramen cecum, passes posteriorly in the midline encased in the superior margin of the falx cerebri, and ends in the *confluens of sinuses* at the internal occipital protuberance. In the parietal region it gives off a number of lateral diverticuli, the *venous lacunae*, into which the *arachnoid villi* or *granulations* project. It receives the superior cerebral veins.
2. The *inferior sagittal sinus* extends along the inferior free margin of the falx cerebri. On reaching the anterior margin of the tentorium cerebelli, it is joined by the *great cerebral vein*, which drains the deep structures of the brain, to form the *straight sinus*.
3. The *straight sinus*, so formed, runs in the attachment of the falx cerebri to the tentorium cerebelli to empty into the confluens of sinuses.
4. The two *transverse sinuses* arise from the confluens of sinuses and pass laterally and anteriorly in a groove in the occipital bone, occupying the attached margin of the tentorium cerebelli. They receive the superior petrosal sinuses, inferior cerebral veins, and cerebellar veins. Most often there is not a true *confluens of sinuses*, but the superior sagittal sinus drains into the right transverse sinus and the straight sinus into the left transverse sinus.
5. At the base of the petrous part of the temporal bone, the transverse sinus on each side curves inferiorly and medially to become the *sigmoid sinus*, which ends at the jugular foramen by emptying into the *internal jugular vein*.
6. The *occipital sinus* lies in the falx cerebelli. It arises near the foramen magnum and ends by emptying into the confluens of sinuses.
7. The *cavernous sinus* is a large irregular space between the periosteal and meningeal layers of the dura. It lies on the side of the body of the sphenoid bone lateral to the sella turcica and extends from the superior orbital fissure to the apex of the petrous part of the temporal bone. The internal carotid artery passes through the center of the sinus accompanied by the abducent nerve (VI). The oculomotor (III) and trochlear (IV) nerves plus the ophthalmic and maxillary divisions of the trigeminal nerve (V) pass anteriorly embedded in its lateral wall. It receives the superior ophthalmic vein at the superior orbital fissure, inferior and middle cerebral veins, and the sphenoparietal sinus. It terminates posteriorly in the superior and inferior petrosal sinuses. It communicates with its fellow on the opposite side via the *intercavernous sinus*.
8. The *sphenoparietal sinus* lies in the dura along the lesser wing of the sphenoid bone and ends in the anterior part of the cavernous sinus.
9. The *intercavernous (circular) sinus* connects the two cavernous sinuses, passing anterior and posterior to the infundibulum of the pituitary gland.
10. The *superior petrosal sinus* lies in the margin of the tentorium cerebelli, which is attached to the superior angle of the petrous part of the temporal bone. It connects the posterior end of the cavernous sinus to the transverse sinus. It receives cerebellar and inferior cerebral veins.
11. The *inferior petrosal sinus* begins at the posterior end of the cavernous sinus, passes through the jugular foramen, and empties into the internal jugular vein. It receives the labyrinthine vein and veins from the medulla, pons, and cerebellum.

***Figure 50* Venous Sinuses of the Dura Mater, as viewed from above (upper plate) and in median section (lower plate)**

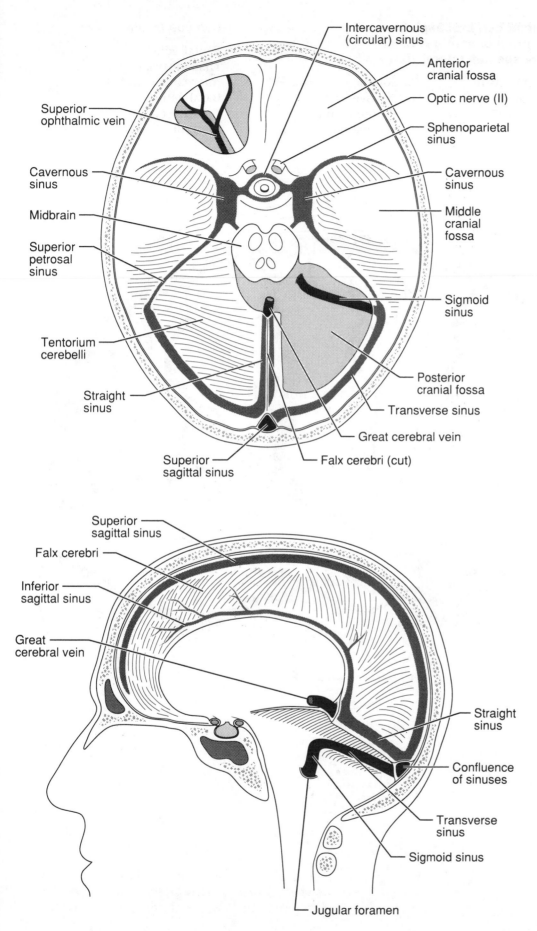

Intercavernous (circular) sinus

Anterior cranial fossa

Optic nerve (II)

Sphenoparietal sinus

Cavernous sinus

Middle cranial fossa

Sigmoid sinus

Posterior cranial fossa

Transverse sinus

Great cerebral vein

Falx cerebri (cut)

Superior ophthalmic vein

Cavernous sinus

Midbrain

Superior petrosal sinus

Tentorium cerebelli

Straight sinus

Superior sagittal sinus

Superior sagittal sinus

Falx cerebri

Inferior sagittal sinus

Great cerebral vein

Straight sinus

Confluence of sinuses

Transverse sinus

Sigmoid sinus

Jugular foramen

Blood Vessels of the Brain   **85**

Figure 51 **Venous phase of cerebral angiogram showing the superficial group of cerebral veins and the dural venous sinuses, left lateral view**

A. Superficial middle cerebral vein
B. Inferior anastomotic vein (Labbé)
C. Superior anastomotic vein (Trolard)
D. Superior cerebral veins
E. Superior sagittal sinus

F. Confluens of sinuses
G. Transverse sinus
H. Sigmoid sinus
I. Internal jugular vein

Can you locate:

Septal vein
Thalamostriate vein
Internal cerebral vein
Basal vein
Great cerebral vein
Straight sinus

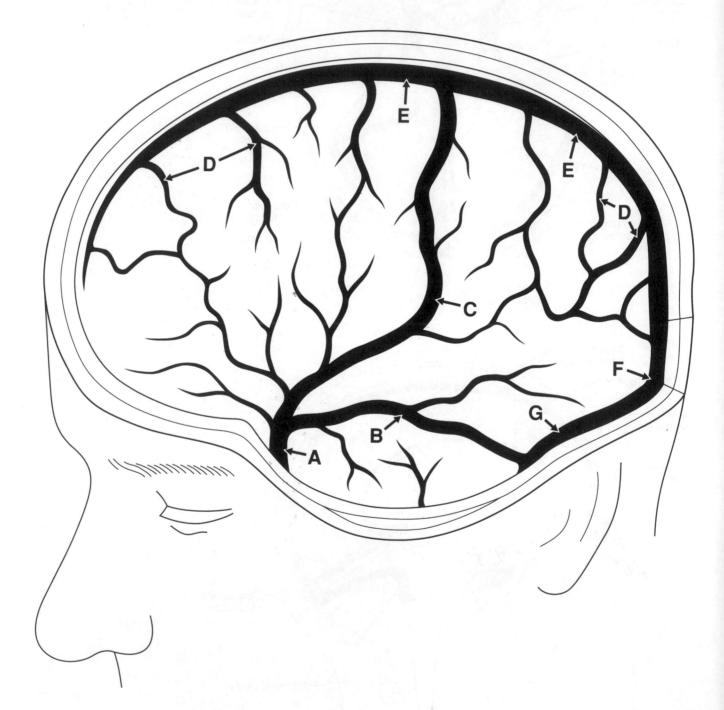

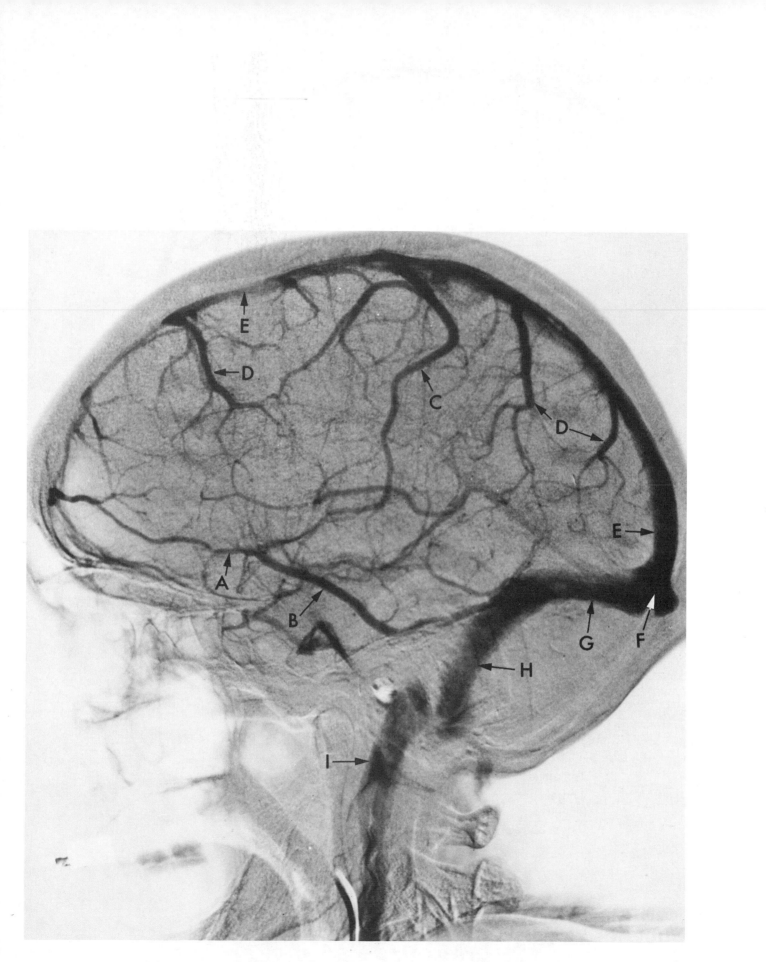

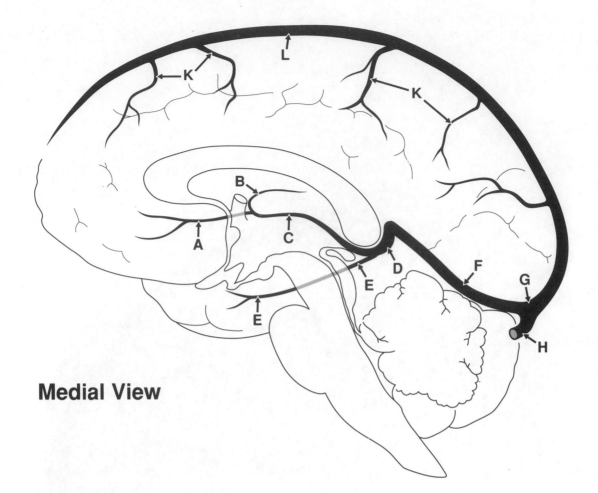

Medial View

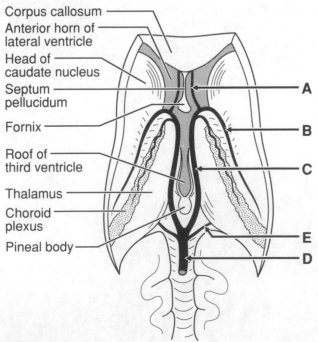

Corpus callosum

Anterior horn of
lateral ventricle

Head of
caudate nucleus

Septum
pellucidum

Fornix

Roof of
third ventricle

Thalamus

Choroid
plexus

Pineal body

A

B

C

E

D

Superior View

Figure 52 Venous phase of cerebral angiogram showing the deep group of cerebral veins and the dural venous sinuses, left lateral view

A. Septal vein
B. Thalamostriate vein
C. Internal cerebral vein
D. Great cerebral vein
E. Basal vein
F. Straight sinus
G. Confluens of sinuses
H. Transverse sinus

I. Sigmoid sinus
J. Internal jugular vein
K. Superior cerebral veins
L. Superior sagittal sinus

Can you locate:

Superficial middle cerebral vein
Superior anastomotic vein

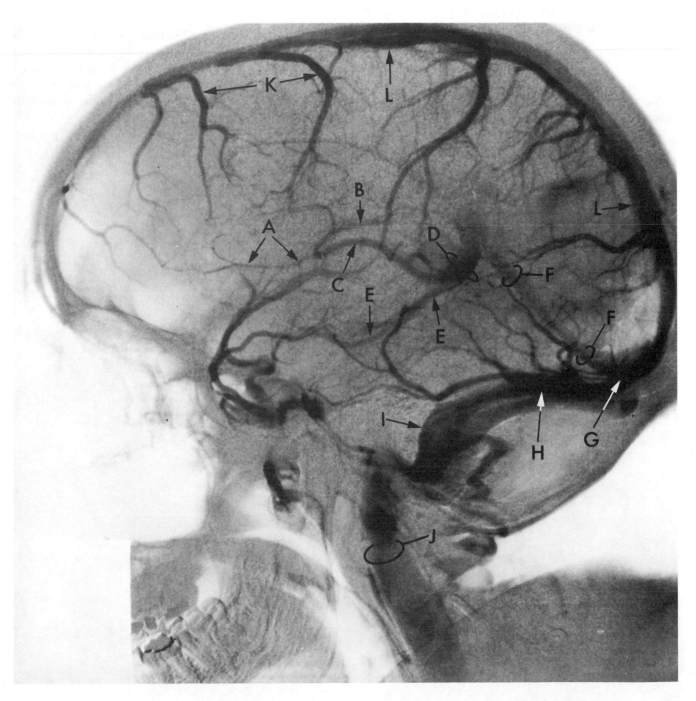

Superficial Cerebral Veins

These veins arise from the cortex and subcortical areas, anastomose freely in the pia mater, and form a number of large veins, which empty into the dural venous sinuses. They include the *superior* and *inferior cerebral veins* and the *superficial middle cerebral vein*. The superficial middle cerebral vein often is connected to the superior sagittal sinus via the large *superior anastomotic vein* (Trolard) and to the transverse sinus via the *inferior anastomotic vein* (Labbé) (Figures 51, 52, and 54).

Deep Cerebral Veins

The deep cerebral veins drain the deep white matter, basal nuclei, and parts of the diencephalon. These veins ultimately terminate in the *internal cerebral veins* and the *great cerebral vein* (Figures 51, 52, and 75).

1. The two *internal cerebral veins* begin in the region of the interventricular foramina by the union of the *septal vein* and the *thalamostriate vein*. They pass posteriorly just lateral to the midline in the tela choroidea of the roof of the third ventricle, enter the quadrigeminal cistern just below the splenium of the corpus callosum, and join with one another to form the *great cerebral vein*.

2. The *great cerebral vein* (Galen), so formed, passes posteriorly beneath the splenium of the corpus callosum, curves upward, and joins the inferior sagittal sinus to form the straight sinus. It receives the two basal veins as well as tributaries from other adjacent structures.

   a. The *basal vein* (Rosenthal) is the most important tributary of the great cerebral vein. It arises near the medial aspect of the anterior temporal lobe, courses posteriorly around the cerebral peduncle near the posterior cerebral artery, and ends in the great cerebral vein near its origin. The basal vein receives the anterior cerebral, deep middle cerebral and inferior striate veins as well as other tributaries from the hypothalamus, midbrain, and adjacent areas.

Blood Vessels
of the Spinal Cord

ARTERIAL SUPPLY TO THE SPINAL CORD

The spinal cord is supplied by the *anterior spinal artery* and the *posterior spinal arteries*. The *anterior spinal artery* begins superiorly by the junction of the two anterior spinal branches of the vertebral arteries. It descends the length of the cord, lying in the anterior median fissure of the spinal cord. It supplies branches to the anterior and lateral gray horns, the central gray matter, and the anterior and lateral funiculi.

The *posterior spinal arteries* also arise as branches from the vertebral arteries. They descend on the cord along the dorsal root entry zone and are somewhat plexiform. They supply the posterior gray horns and the posterior funiculi.

Both the anterior and posterior spinal arteries are reinforced segmentally. The *spinal rami* of the vertebral, intercostal, lumbar, and lateral sacral arteries accompany the spinal nerves through the intervertebral foramina and divide into *anterior* and *posterior radicular arteries*, which contribute to the anterior and posterior spinal arteries respectively. Not all spinal nerves are accompanied by radicular arteries, and probably only eight to ten anterior and ten to fifteen posterior radicular arteries are of significance. A *great anterior radicular artery* (Adamkiewicz) is recognized as providing a ma-jor contribution to the anterior spinal artery in the lower thoracic or upper lumbar region (Figure 53).

VENOUS RETURN FROM THE SPINAL CORD

The veins of the spinal cord resemble the corresponding arteries in their general distribution and form a plexiform arrangement in the pia mater. There usually are three large channels in this plexus anteriorly and three channels posteriorly (the *anterior* and *posterior spinal veins*), which drain into *anterior* and *posterior radicular veins*. These radicular veins join with the *anterior* and *posterior internal venous plexus* in the epidural space to form the *intervertebral veins*, which exit with the spinal nerves and arteries through the intervertebral foramina to end in the vertebral, intercostal, lumbar, and lateral sacral veins. The *internal vertebral venous plexuses* also communicate with the *anterior external venous plexus*, via the *basivertebral veins* in the body of the vertebrae, and with the *posterior external venous plexus*. These external plexuses are located on the anterolateral aspect of the vertebral bodies and on the posterior aspect of the laminae of the vertebrae (Figure 53).

Figure 53 Arterial and venous supply to the spinal cord

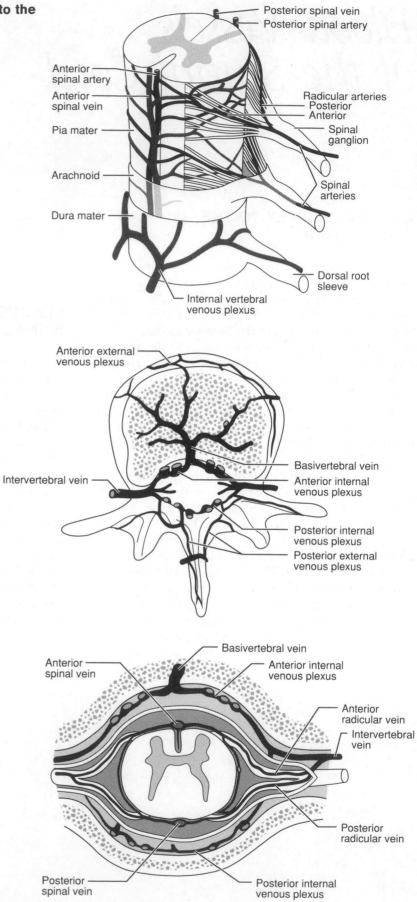

Posterior spinal vein
Posterior spinal artery

Anterior spinal artery

Anterior spinal vein

Pia mater

Arachnoid

Dura mater

Radicular arteries
Posterior
Anterior

Spinal ganglion

Spinal arteries

Dorsal root sleeve

Internal vertebral venous plexus

Anterior external venous plexus

Intervertebral vein

Basivertebral vein

Anterior internal venous plexus

Posterior internal venous plexus

Posterior external venous plexus

Basivertebral vein

Anterior spinal vein

Anterior internal venous plexus

Anterior radicular vein

Intervertebral vein

Posterior radicular vein

Posterior spinal vein

Posterior internal venous plexus

Part Four
Atlas of the Brain and Spinal Cord

SURFACE VIEWS OF THE BRAIN

Figure 54 **Lateral view of the brain, arachnoid and pia mater intact (×1)**

A. Frontal pole of cerebral hemisphere
B. Frontal lobe
C. Parietal lobe
D. Occipital lobe
E. Occipital pole
F. Temporal pole
G. Temporal lobe
H. Small piece of dura mater
I. Superficial cerebral veins emptying into the superior sagittal sinus
J. Cerebellum
K. Pons
L. Medulla

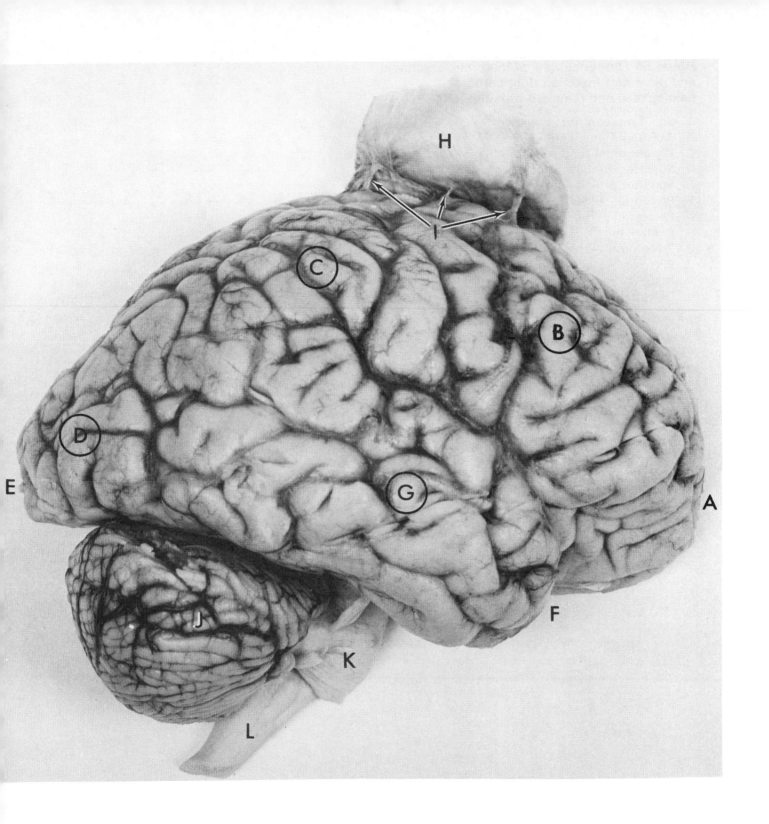

Figure 55 **Superior view of the brain, arachnoid and pia mater intact on right cerebral hemisphere and removed from the left (×1)**

A. Small piece of dura mater
B. Arachnoid granulations
C. Longitudinal cerebral fissure
D. Superior frontal gyrus
E. Superior frontal sulcus
F. Precentral sulcus
G. Precentral gyrus
H. Central sulcus
I. Postcentral gyrus
J. Postcentral sulcus
K. Marginal ramus of cingulate sulcus
L. Occipital lobe

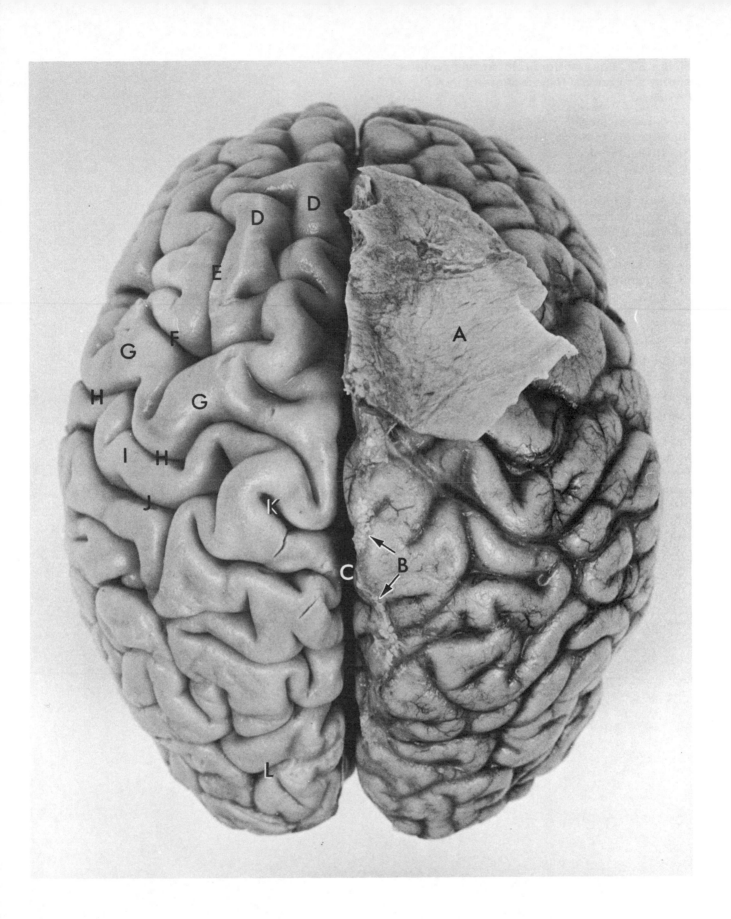

Figure 56 Base of the brain showing arterial supply and cranial nerves. Anteroinferior view (×1.5)

A. Olfactory sulcus
B. Olfactory bulb
C. Olfactory tract
D. Anterior cerebral artery (notice difference in size between right and left)
E. Anterior communicating artery
F. Posterior cerebral artery
G. Oculomotor nerve (III)
H. Superior cerebellar artery (double on the right)
 I. Basilar artery
 J. Trigeminal nerve (V)
K. Facial nerve (VII)
L. Vestibulocochlear nerve (VIII)
M. Glossopharyngeal (IX), vagus (X), and cranial part of accessory (XI) nerves
N. Vertebral artery
O. Posterior inferior cerebellar artery
P. Cut surface of temporal lobe

Can you locate:

Internal carotid artery
Middle cerebral artery
Posterior communicating artery
Anterior inferior cerebellar artery
Inferior horn of lateral ventricle
Optic nerve
Optic chiasma

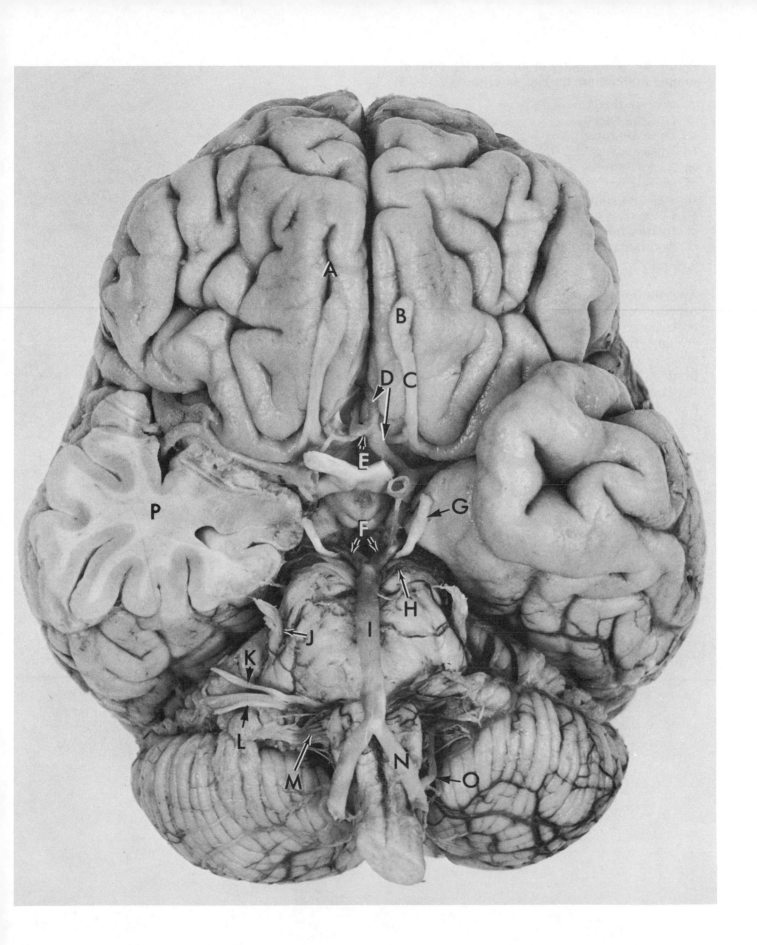

Figure 57 Base of the brain showing arterial supply and cranial nerves. Inferior view (×1.5)

A. Longitudinal cerebral fissure
B. Optic nerve (II)
C. Optic chiasma
D. Optic tract
E. Internal carotid artery
F. Middle cerebral artery (in lateral sulcus)
G. Posterior communicating artery
H. Cut surface of temporal lobe
 I. Inferior horn of lateral ventricle
 J. Anterior inferior cerebellar artery

Can you locate:

Anterior cerebral arteries
Anterior communicating artery
Posterior cerebral artery
Oculomotor nerve
Superior cerebellar artery
Basilar artery
Vertebral artery
Posterior inferior cerebellar artery
Facial nerve
Vestibulocochlear nerve
Flocculus of cerebellum
Choroid plexus of lateral recess of fourth ventricle
    (in cerebellopontine angle)
Cerebellar hemisphere
Olfactory bulb and tract
Medial and lateral olfactory striae
Trigeminal nerve
Tuber cinereum
Mamillary bodies

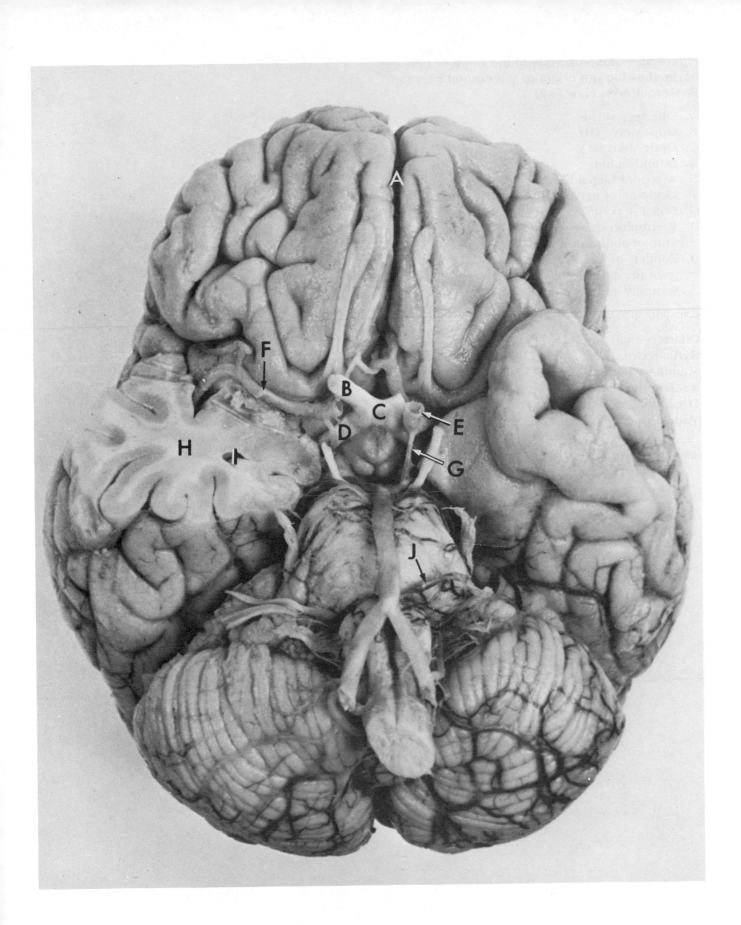

Figure 58 **Close-up view of the base of the brain showing the origin of the cranial nerves. Posteroinferior view (×2)**

A. Olfactory sulcus
B. Optic nerve (II)
C. Optic chiasma
D. Infundibulum
E. Arachnoid (spanning a sulcus)
F. Oculomotor nerve (III)
G. Facial nerve (VII)
H. Vestibulocochlear nerve (VIII)
I. Stub of abducent nerve (VI)
J. Rootlets of hypoglossal nerve (XII) (emerging from the *anterolateral sulcus* between the *pyramid* ventrally and the *olive* dorsally)

Can you locate:

Olfactory bulb and tract
Gyrus rectus
Mamillary bodies
Basilar artery
Trigeminal nerve
Middle cerebellar peduncle

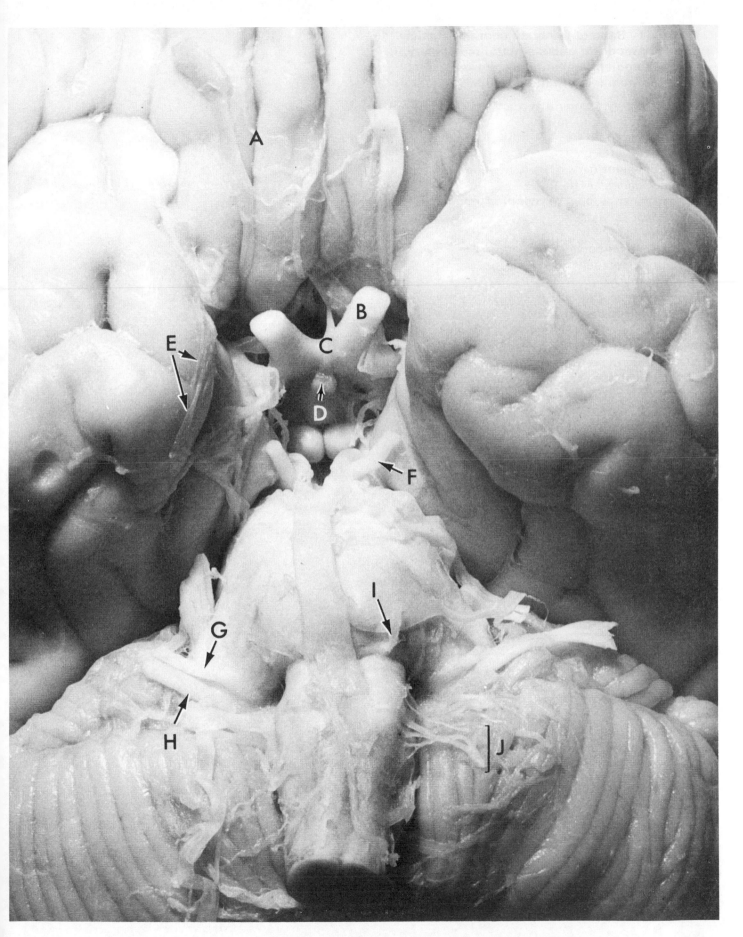

Figure 59 Base of the brain showing cranial nerves. Arachnoid and pia mater intact on right cerebral and cerebellar hemispheres and removed from the left. Inferior view (×1.5)

A. Straight gyrus (gyrus rectus)
B. Orbital gyri and sulci
C. Olfactory bulb
D. Olfactory tract
E. Oculomotor nerve (III) (emerging from *interpeduncular fossa*)
F. Trochlear nerve (IV) (winding around left *cerebral peduncle*)
G. Pons
H. Trigeminal nerve (V)
I. Middle cerebellar peduncle
J. Facial nerve (VII)
K. Vestibulocochlear nerve (VIII)
L. Hypoglossal nerve (XII)
M. Flocculus of cerebellum
N. Cerebellar hemisphere
O. Choroid plexus of lateral recess of fourth ventricle (in cerebellopontine angle)

Can you locate:

Longitudinal cerebral fissure
Mamillary bodies
Posterior perforated substance
Pyramid and olive of medulla
Uncus
Parahippocampal gyrus
Rhinal sulcus

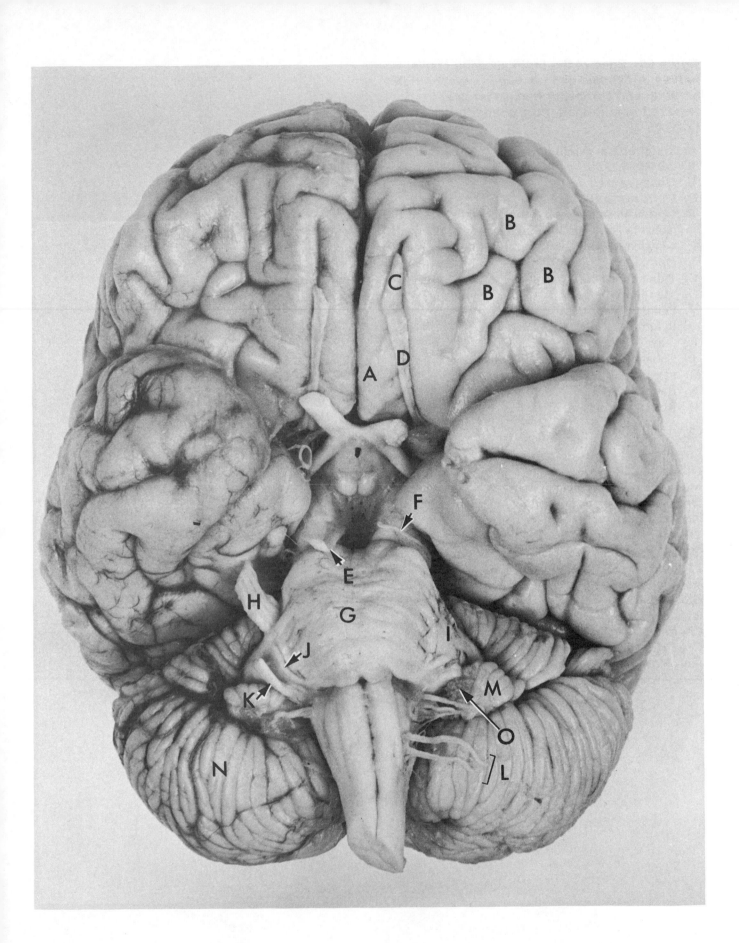

Figure 60 Base of the brain showing cranial nerves. Arachnoid and pia mater intact on right cerebral and cerebellar hemispheres and removed from the left. Posteroinferior view (×1.5)

A. Longitudinal cerebral fissure
B. Olfactory bulb
C. Olfactory tract
D. Optic nerve (II)
E. Optic chiasma (the opening directly behind the chiasma is the infundibular recess of the third ventricle within the infundibulum)
F. Optic tract
G. Tuber cinereum
H. Mamillary body
I. Pons
J. Pyramid
K. Olive
L. Collateral sulcus
M. Parahippocampal gyrus
N. Uncus
O. Rhinal sulcus

Can you locate:

Straight gyrus (gyrus rectus)
Orbital gyri and sulci
Medial and lateral olfactory striae
Anterior and posterior perforated substances
Oculomotor nerve
Trigeminal nerve
Middle cerebellar peduncle
Facial nerve
Vestibulocochlear nerve
Glossopharyngeal, vagus, and accessory nerves
Hypoglossal nerve
Choroid plexus of lateral recess of fourth ventricle
Cerebellopontine angle (cistern)
Flocculus of cerebellum
Cerebellar hemisphere

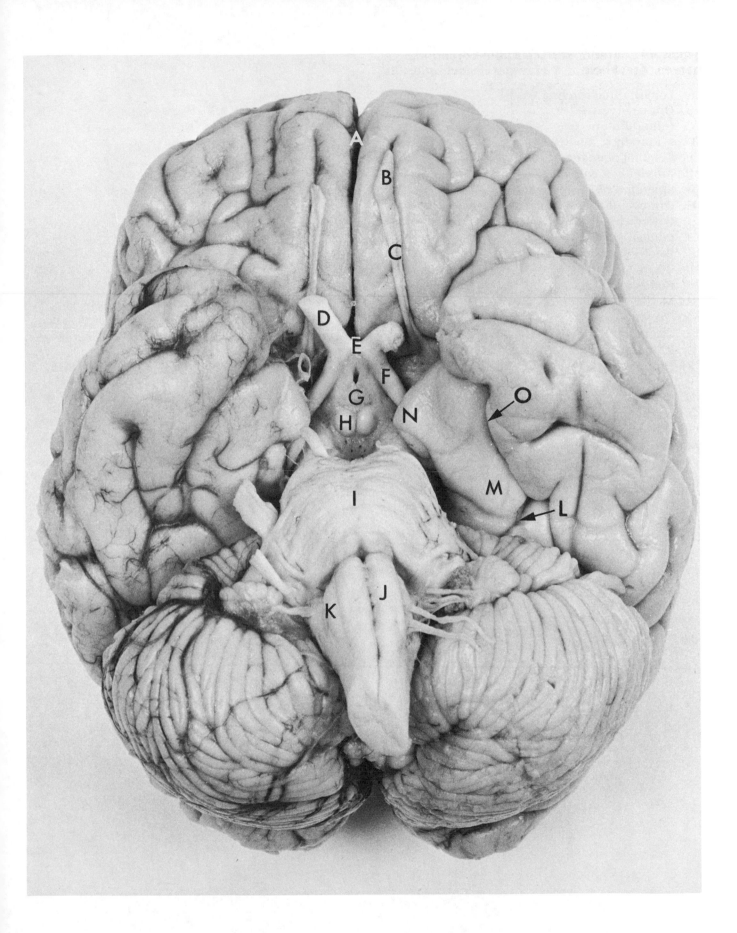

Figure 61 Inferior surface of the cerebrum, brain stem removed. Posteroinferior view (×1.5)

A. Longitudinal cerebral fissure
B. Optic nerve (II)
C. Infundibulum
D. Midbrain (cut surface)
E. Cerebral aqueduct
F. Inferior colliculus
G. Splenium of corpus callosum
H. Isthmus of cingulate gyrus
I. Calcarine sulcus
J. Lingual gyrus
K. Parahippocampal gyrus
L. Uncus
M. Collateral sulcus
N. Medial occipitotemporal gyrus
O. Occipitotemporal sulcus
P. Lateral occipitotemporal gyrus
Q. Rhinal sulcus
R. Hippocampal sulcus

Can you locate:

Olfactory bulb and tract
Optic chiasma and tract
Mamillary bodies
Oculomotor nerve

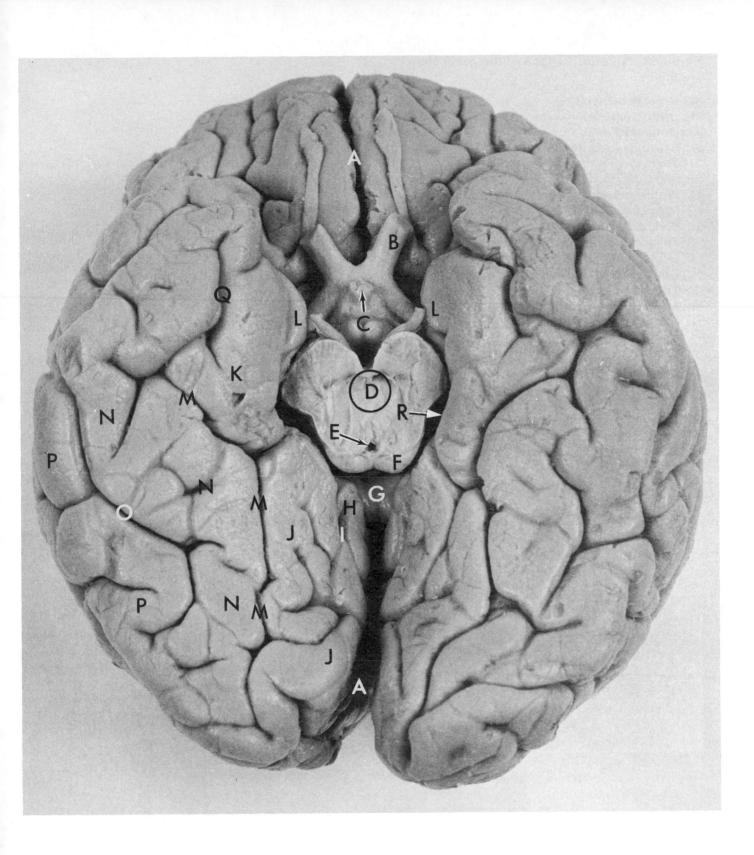

Figure 62 Anterior surface of the brain stem (×2.25)

A. Optic nerve (II)
B. Optic chiasma
C. Optic tract
D. Lateral geniculate body
E. Tuber cinereum
F. Mamillary body
G. Posterior perforated substance in floor of *interpeduncular fossa*
H. Cerebral peduncle
I. Trochlear nerve (IV)
J. Oculomotor nerve (III)
K. Basilar sulcus of the pons
L. Trigeminal nerve (V)
M. Middle cerebellar peduncle
N. Abducent nerve (VI)
O. Facial nerve (VII)
P. Vestibulocochlear nerve (VIII)
Q. Glossopharyngeal (IX) and vagus (X) nerves
R. Pyramid of medulla
S. Olive
T. Hypoglossal nerve (XII)
U. Spinal part of the accessory nerve (XI)

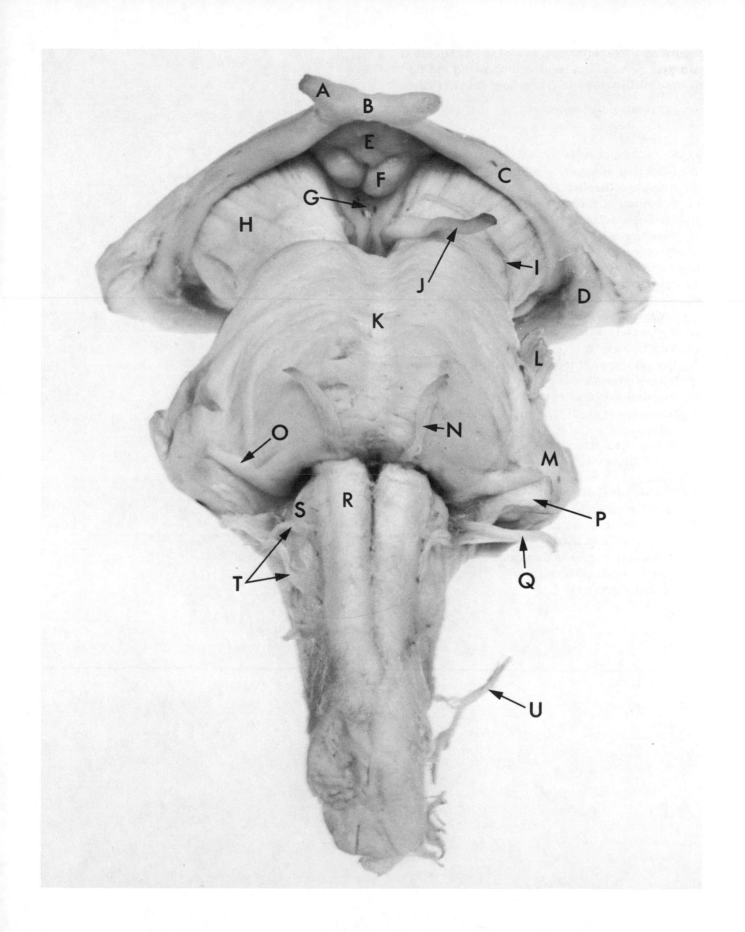

Figure 63 **Posterior surface of the brain stem with the cerebellum removed showing the floor of the fourth ventricle (rhomboid fossa) (×2)**

A. Pulvinar of thalamus
B. Pineal body
C. Habenula
D. Superior colliculus
E. Brachium of superior colliculus
F. Inferior colliculus
G. Brachium of inferior colliculus
H. Medial geniculate body
I. Superior medullary velum
J. Trochlear nerve (IV)
K. Superior cerebellar peduncle
L. Middle cerebellar peduncle
M. Medial eminence (bounded medially by the *median sulcus*)
N. Facial colliculus
O. Vestibular area
P. Lateral recess of fourth ventricle overlying the *inferior cerebellar peduncle*
Q. Vestibulocochlear nerve (VIII)
R. Glossopharyngeal (IX) and part of vagus (X) nerves
S. Hypoglossal trigone
T. Vagal trigone
U. Obex
V. Gracile tubercle
W. Cuneate tubercle
X. Fasciculus gracilis (bounded medially by the *posterior median sulcus*)
Y. Fasciculus cuneatus (bounded medially by the *posterior intermediate sulcus*)
Z. C_2 dorsal rootlets

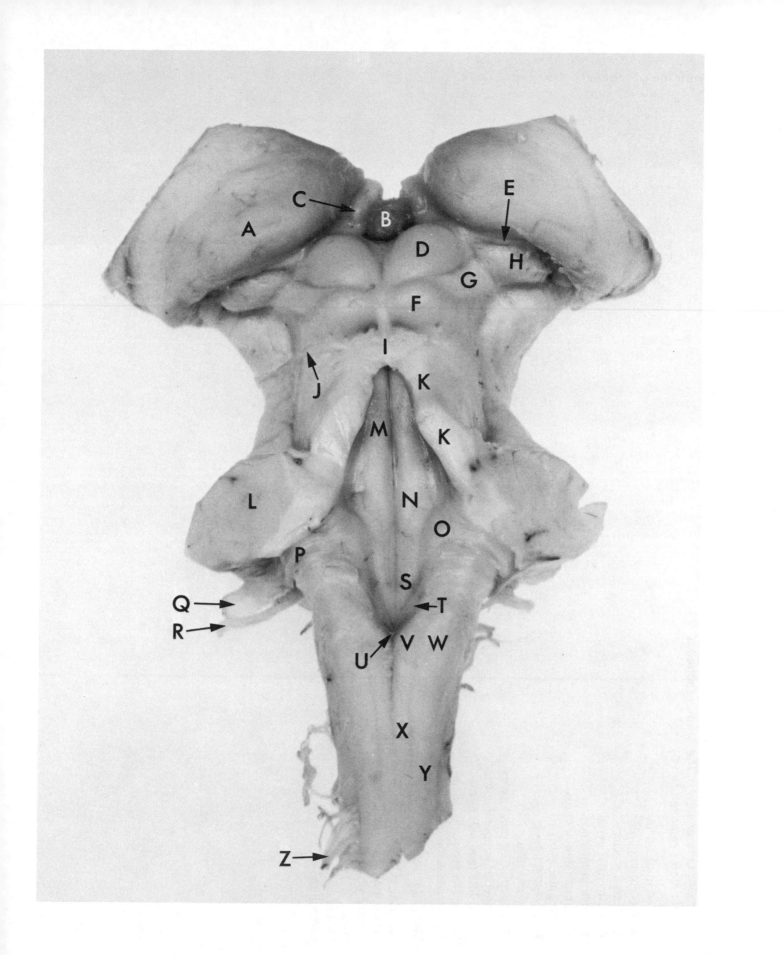

Figure 64 **Lateral view of the brain, arachnoid and pia mater removed (×1.5)**

A. Precentral sulcus
B. Precentral gyrus
C. Central sulcus
D. Postcentral gyrus
E. Postcentral sulcus
F. Supramarginal gyrus
G. Angular gyrus
H. Occipital lobe
I. Lateral sulcus
J. Superior temporal gyrus
K. Superior temporal sulcus
L. Middle temporal gyrus
M. Inferior temporal sulcus
N. Inferior temporal gyrus

Can you locate:

Superior, middle, and inferior frontal gyri
Superior and inferior frontal sulci
Frontal, occipital, and temporal poles
Pons
Medulla
Cerebellum

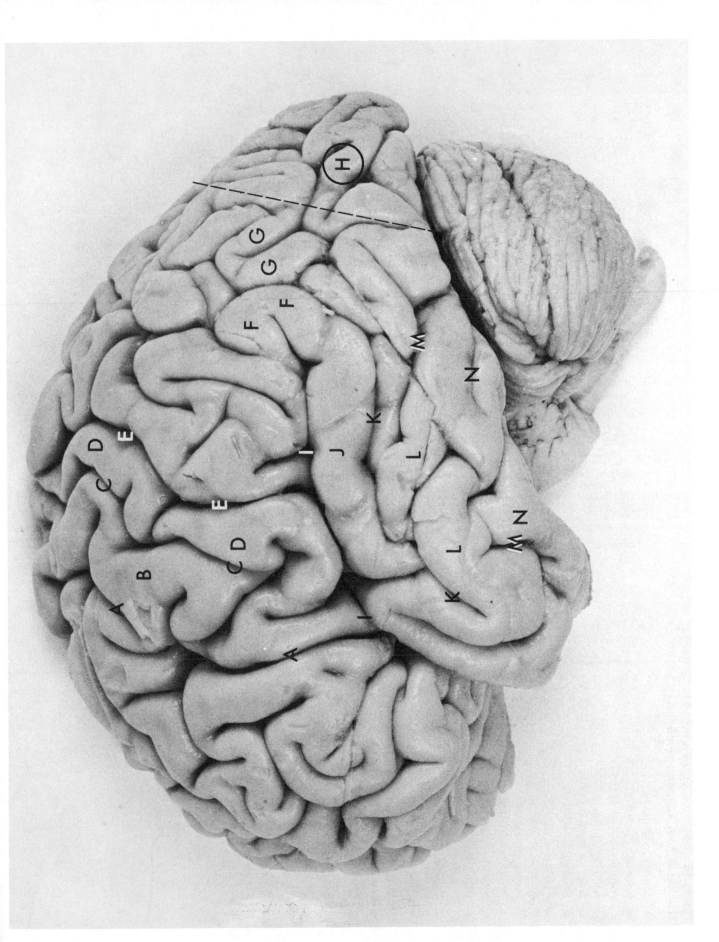

Figure 65 **Superolateral view of the brain, arachnoid and pia mater removed (×1.5)**

A. Superior frontal gyrus
B. Superior frontal sulcus
C. Middle frontal gyrus
D. Inferior frontal sulcus
E. Inferior frontal gyrus
F. Precentral sulcus
G. Precentral gyrus
H. Central sulcus
I. Postcentral gyrus
J. Postcentral sulcus
K. Superior parietal lobule
L. Intraparietal sulcus
M. Inferior parietal lobule
N. Cerebellum

Can you locate:

Marginal ramus of cingulate sulcus
Supramarginal and angular gyri
Lateral sulcus
Superior temporal gyrus and sulcus
Occipital lobe

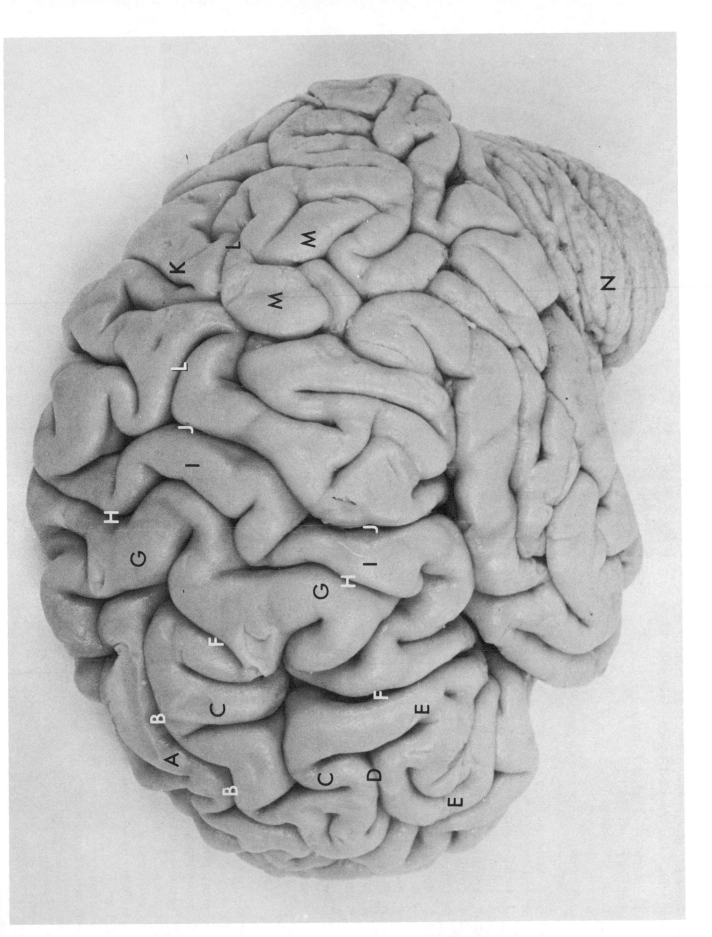

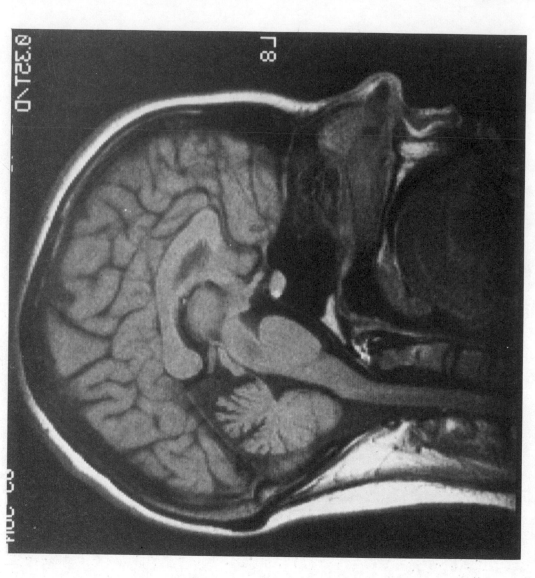

Normal T1-weighted MRI scan

Figure 66 **Medial view of the brain, arachnoid and pia mater removed. Median section (×1.5)**

A. Straight gyrus (gyrus rectus)
B. Paraterminal gyrus
C. Subcallosal area
D. Cingulate gyrus
E. Cingulate sulcus (and its marginal ramus)
F. Paracentral lobule
G. Central sulcus
H. Precuneus
I. Parieto-occipital sulcus
J. Calcarine sulcus
K. Splenium of corpus callosum
L. Trunk of corpus callosum
M. Genu of corpus callosum
N. Rostrum of corpus callosum
O. Septum pellucidum
P. Body of fornix
Q. Choroid plexus of lateral ventricle
R. Pineal body
S. Interthalamic adhesion
T. Anterior commissure
U. Cerebral aqueduct
V. Superior medullary velum
W. Fourth ventricle

Can you locate:

Medial frontal gyrus
Cuneus
Lingual gyrus
Interventricular foramen
Thalamus and hypothalamus
Optic nerve and chiasma
Optic recess of third ventricle
Midbrain (cerebral peduncle and tectum)
Pons
Medulla
Posterior commissure

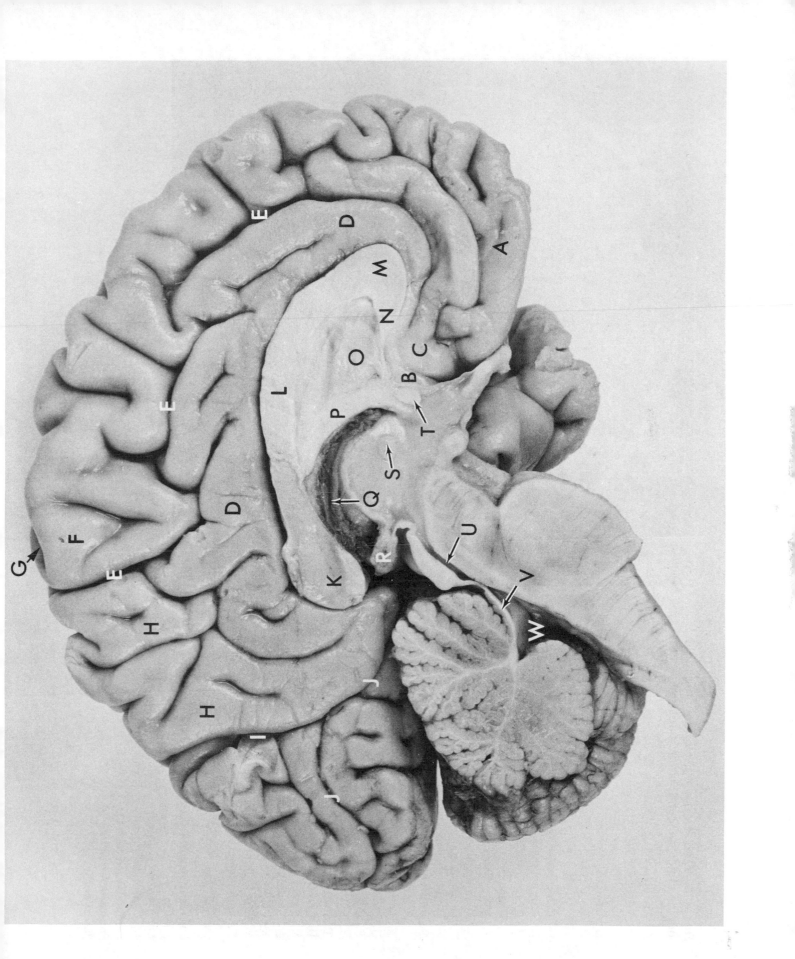

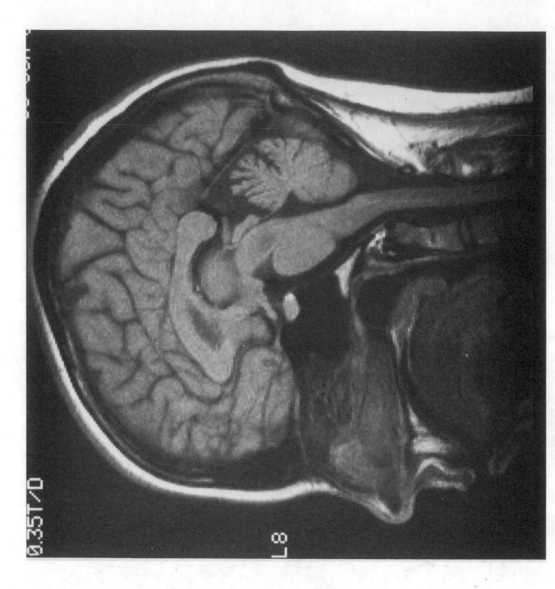

0.35T/0

L8

Normal T1-weighted MRI scan

Figure 67 **Medial view of the brain, arachnoid and pia mater removed. Median section (×1.5)**

A. Medial frontal gyrus
B. Cingulate sulcus
C. Cingulate gyrus
D. Isthmus of cingulate gyrus
E. Parieto-occipital sulcus
F. Cuneus
G. Calcarine sulcus
H. Lingual gyrus
I. Interventricular foramen
J. Thalamus
K. Hypothalamic sulcus (position of)
L. Hypothalamus
M. Optic recess of third ventricle
N. Optic chiasma
O. Infundibulum and infundibular recess of third ventricle
P. Tuber cinereum
Q. Mamillary body
R. Posterior commissure
S. Superior colliculus
T. Inferior colliculus
U. Cerebral peduncle of midbrain
V. Pons (anterior or basilar part)
W. Medulla
X. Cerebellum (vermis)
Y. Cerebellum (hemisphere)
Z. Pons (tegmentum or posterior part)

Can you locate:

Corpus callosum (rostrum, genu, trunk, splenium)
Fornix
Anterior commissure
Pineal recess of third ventricle
Cerebral aqueduct
Fourth ventricle
Pineal body

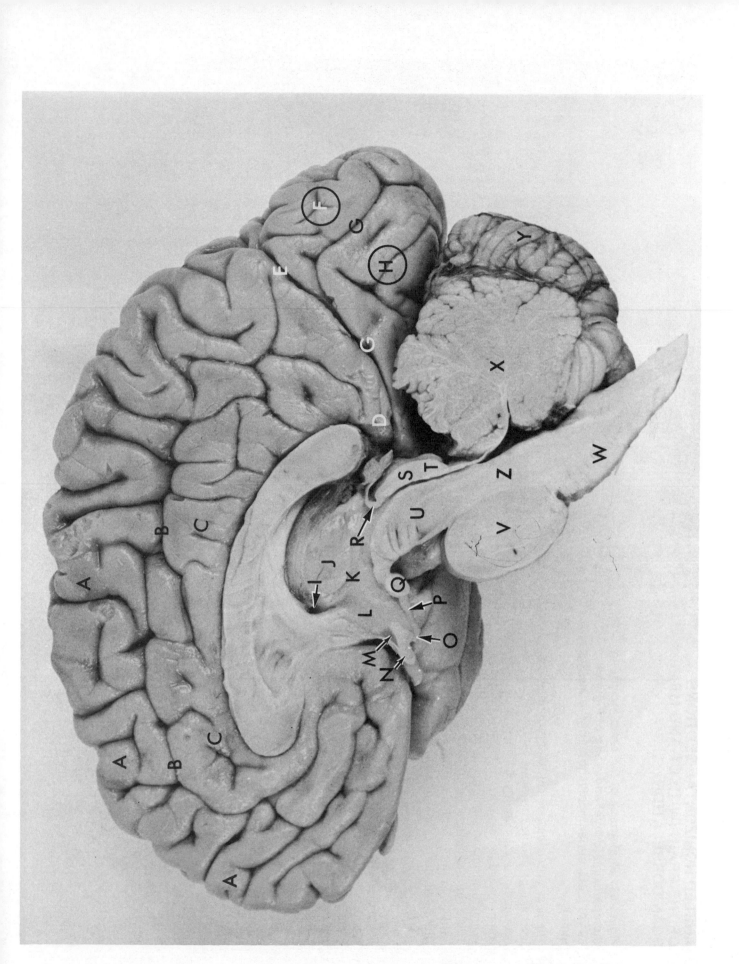

ANGLED HORIZONTAL SECTIONS OF THE BRAIN (WITH CT AND MRI SCAN CORRELATION)

Figure 68 **Photograph of the brain indicating the approximate level and plane of Figures 69–79 (LeMasurier modification of the Mulligan stain)**

The next 11 sections are cut to approximate, in level and plane, the cuts made by the neuroradiological techniques known as computerized tomography, or CT scanning, and magnetic resonance imaging, or MRI scanning. These cuts are made at an angle of approximately 15 degrees to the orbitomeatal line and are illustrated on the photograph on the next page.

It is hoped that the student will be able to identify, on the normal MRI and CT scans, many of the anatomical structures that are labeled on the brain sections. In addition, the student should attempt to correlate the position of other important structures, not visible on the scans, by using the relationships that are clearly visible on the brain sections.

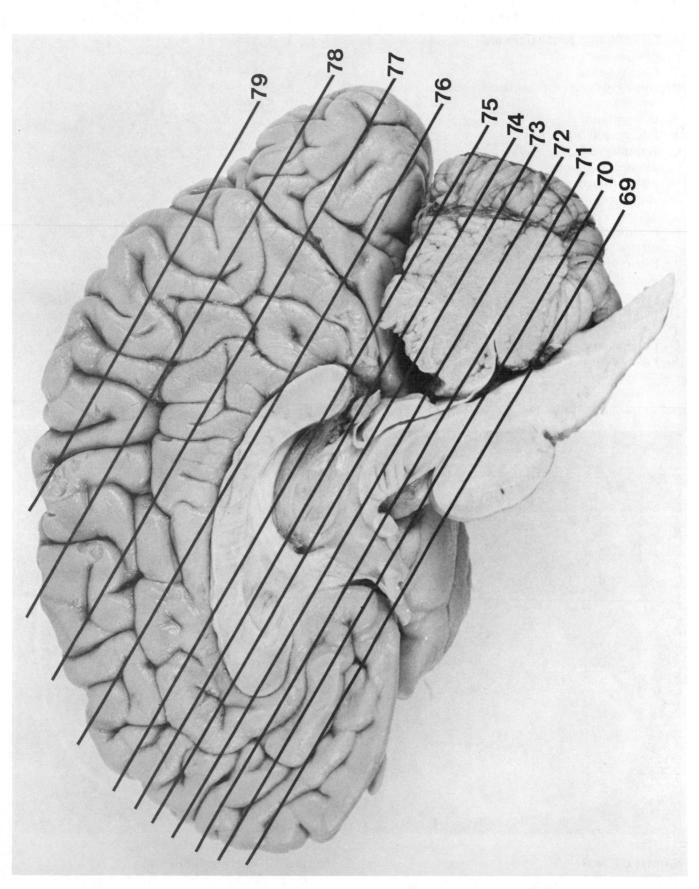

Figure 69 Angled horizontal section of the brain passing through the cerebellum, pons, infundibulum, and optic chiasma (×1.25)

A. Longitudinal cerebral fissure
B. Frontal lobe
C. Lateral sulcus
D. Optic chiasma (surrounded by the chiasmatic cistern)
E. Infundibulum
F. Middle cerebral artery
G. Temporal lobe
H. Amygdaloid body
I. Inferior horn of lateral ventricle
J. Hippocampus (hippocampal digitations, head, or pes)
K. Position of interpeduncular cistern or sella turcica (depending on level of the section)
L. Prepontine cistern
M. Pons (just above level of trigeminal nerves)
N. Fourth ventricle
O. Cerebellar vermis
P. Cerebellar hemisphere
Q. Cerebellomedullary cistern (cisterna magna)
R. Position of pertrous part of temporal bone (on CT scan)

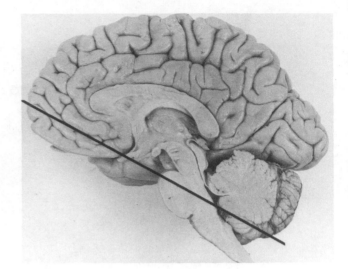

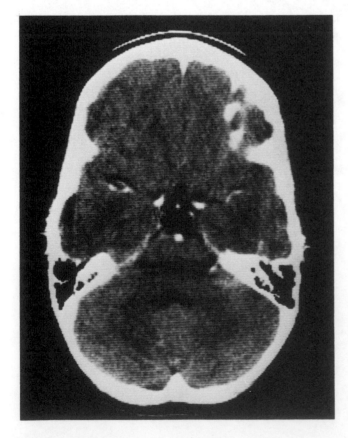

Normal CT scan

Normal T1-weighted MRI scan

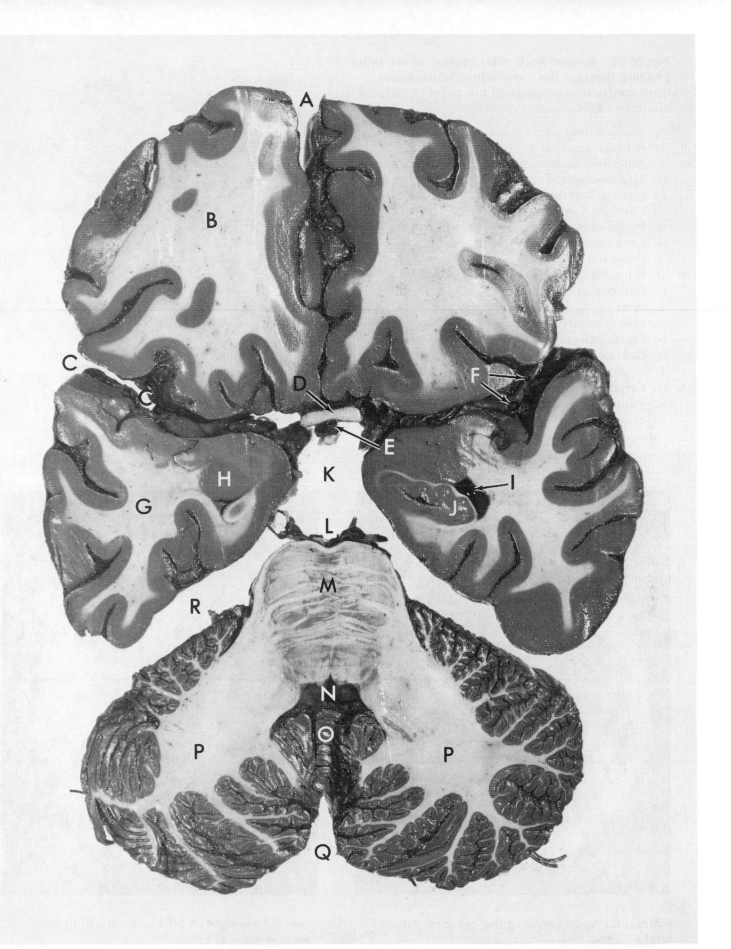

Figure 70 Angled horizontal section of the brain passing through the cerebellum, pons, lower third ventricle, and parts of the cerebral arterial circle (×1.25)

A. Longitudinal cerebral fissure
B. Anterior cerebral artery
C. Anterior communicating artery
D. Middle cerebral artery (within the *lateral sulcus*)
E. Internal carotid artery
F. Posterior communicating artery
G. Posterior cerebral artery
H. Optic recess of third ventricle
I. Optic tract
J. Infundibular recess of third ventricle
K. Interpeduncular cistern
L. Pons
M. Fourth ventricle
N. Cerebellar vermis
O. Dentate nucleus of cerebellum
P. Cerebellar hemisphere
Q. Cerebellomedullary cistern (cisterna magna)
R. Frontal lobe
S. Tip of anterior horn of lateral ventricle

T. Head of caudate nucleus
U. Putamen
V. Lateral sulcus (with branches of middle cerebral artery in it)
W. Temporal lobe
X. Inferior horn of lateral ventricle
Y. Hippocampus

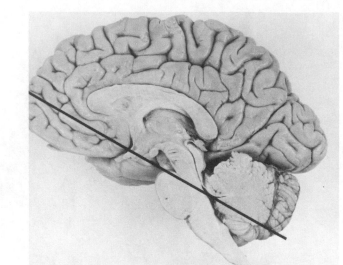

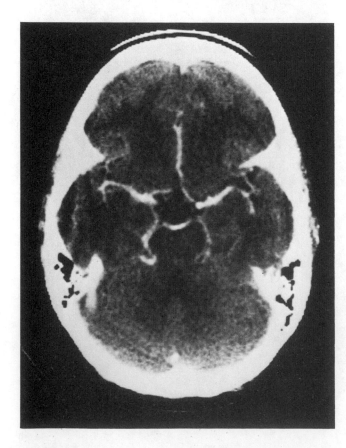

Normal CT scan showing the cerebral arterial circle

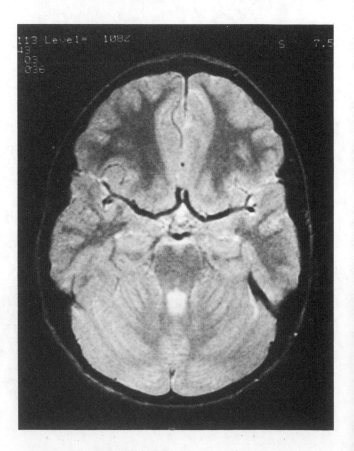

Normal T2-weighted MRI scan showing the cerebral arterial circle

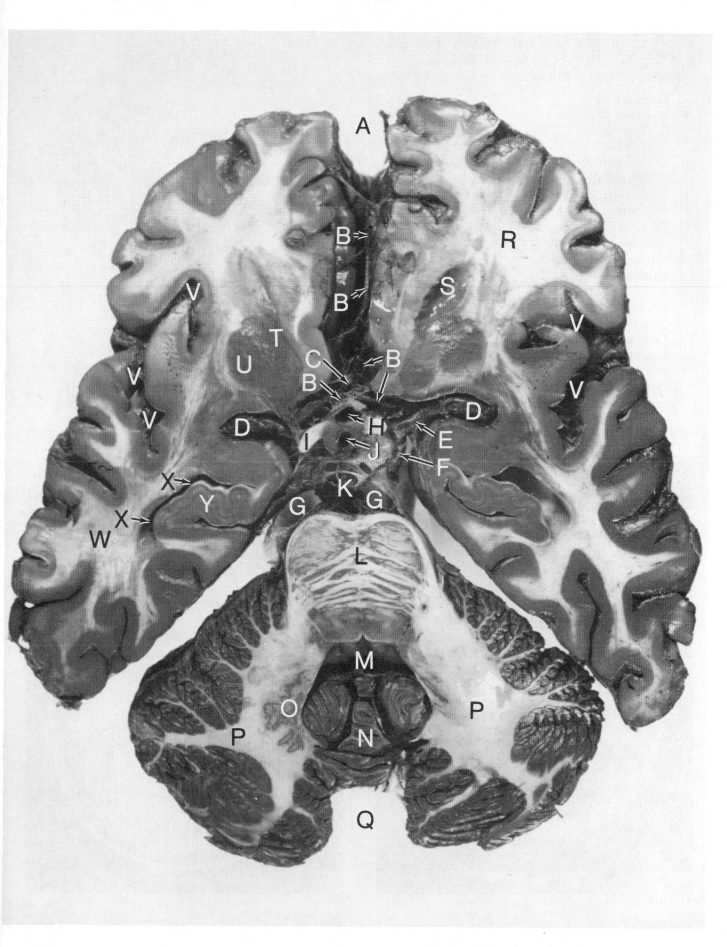

Figure 71 Angled horizontal section of the brain passing through the cerebellum, midbrain, mamillary bodies, and lamina terminalis (×1.25)

A. Frontal lobe
B. Rostrum of corpus callosum
C. Anterior cerebral arteries (running in the *longitudinal cerebral fissure*)
D. Lamina terminalis (*cistern of the lamina terminalis* is just anterior to this structure)
E. Third ventricle (inferior part)
F. Hypothalamus
G. Column of fornix (entering mamillary body)
H. Mamillary body
I. Interpeduncular cistern
J. Optic tract
K. Ambient cistern
L. Midbrain
M. Fourth ventricle
N. Cerebellar vermis
O. Cerebellar hemisphere
P. Dentate nucleus of cerebellum
Q. Dentatorubrothalamic tract (leaving the dentate nucleus and ascending, via the *superior cerebellar peduncle*, to the midbrain)
R. Temporal lobe

S. Inferior horn of lateral ventricle
T. Hippocampus
U. Putamen of lentiform nucleus
V. Head of caudate nucleus
W. Anterior limb of internal capsule
X. Tip of anterior horn of lateral ventricle
Y. Lateral sulcus (with branches of middle cerebral artery in it)

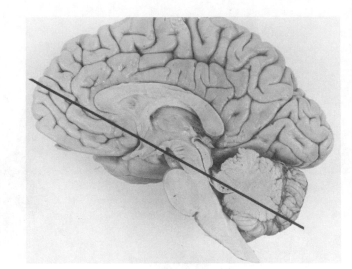

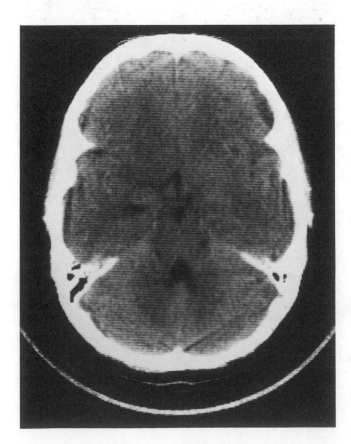

Normal CT scan

Normal T1-weighted MRI scan

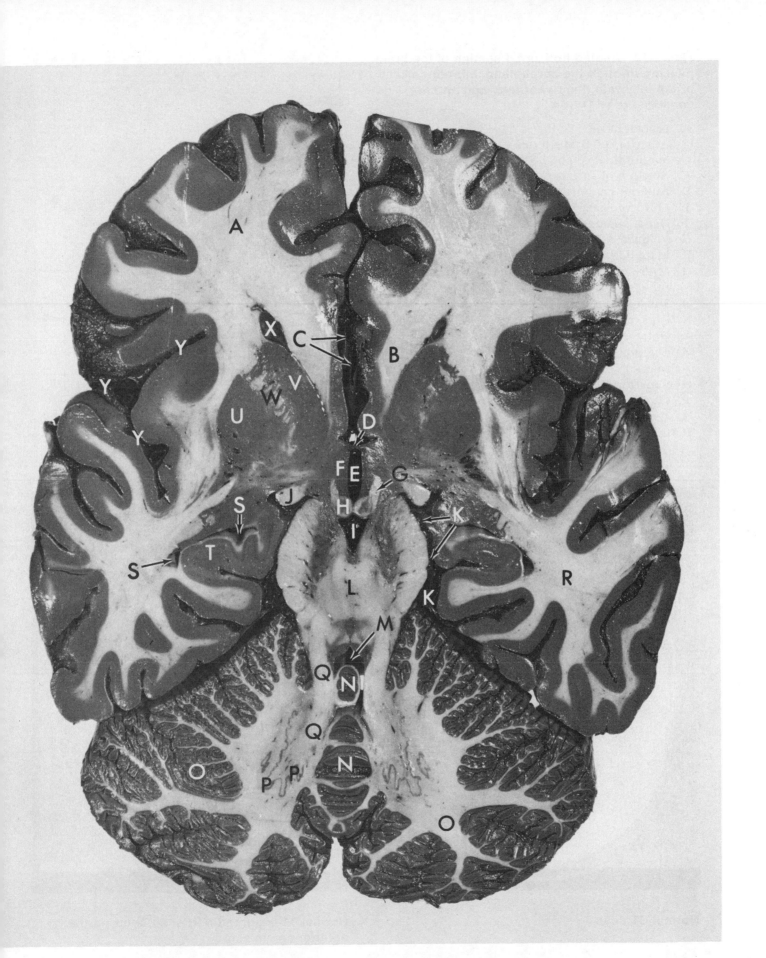

Figure 72 **Angled horizontal section of the brain passing through the cerebellum, inferior colliculi of the midbrain, third ventricle, and anterior commissure (×1)**

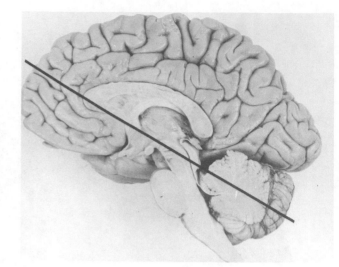

A. Frontal lobe
B. Anterior cerebral arteries (within the longitudinal cerebral fissure)
C. Rostrum of corpus callosum
D. Anterior commissure
E. Third ventricle
F. Hypothalamus
G. Column of fornix
H. Mamillothalamic tract
I. Midbrain (showing the inferior aspect of the *red nuclei*)
J. Substantia nigra
K. Crus cerebri
L. Optic tract
M. Cerebral aqueduct
N. Inferior colliculus
O. Superior (or quadrigeminal) cistern
P. Cerebellum
Q. Temporal lobe
R. Inferior horn of lateral ventricle

S. Hippocampus
T. Tail of caudate nucleus
U. Putamen
V. Anterior limb of internal capsule (white matter)
W. Head of caudate nucleus

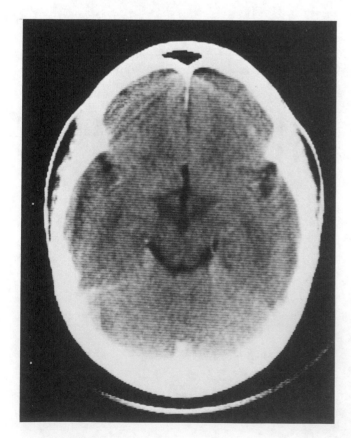

Normal CT scan

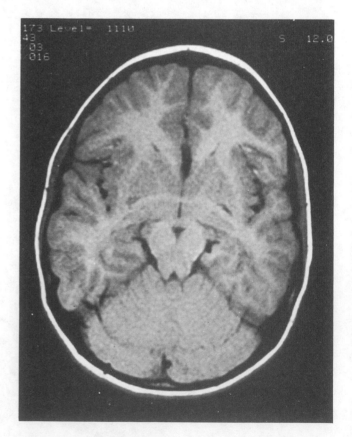

Normal T1-weighted MRI scan showing the anterior commissure

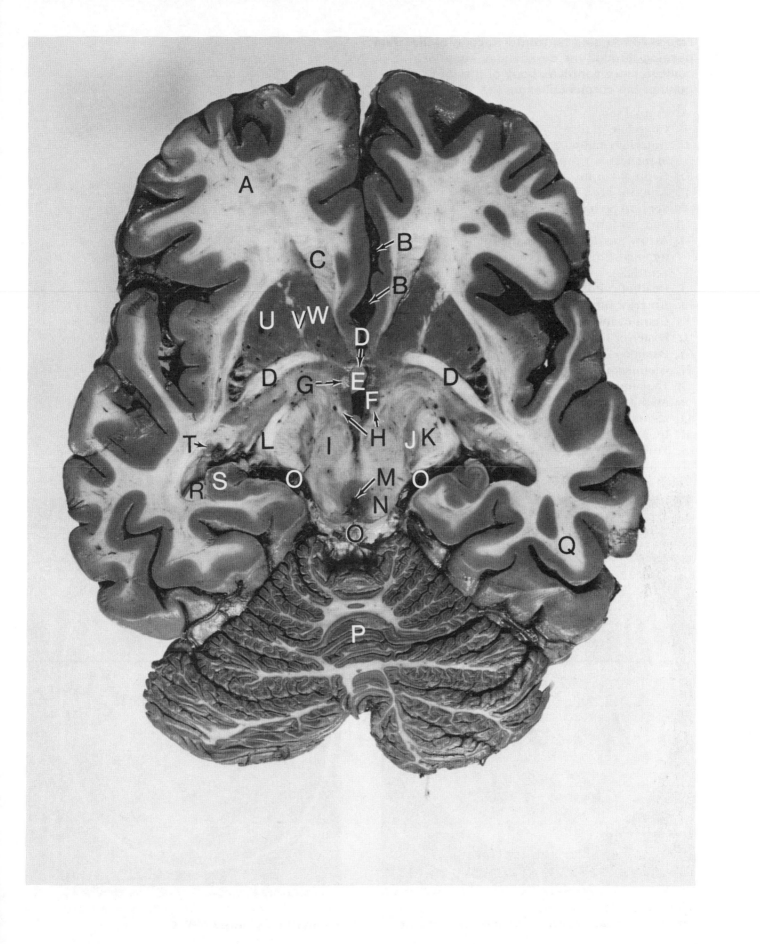

Figure 73 Angled horizontal section of the brain passing through the cerebellum, superior colliculi, third ventricle, body of the fornix, and genu of the corpus callosum (×1.25)

A. Frontal lobe
B. Cingulate gyrus
C. Anterior cerebral arteries (pericallosal branches)
D. Genu of corpus callosum
E. Anterior horn of lateral ventricle
F. Septum pellucidum
G. Body of fornix
H. Arrow passing through the interventricular foramen (from lateral ventricle to third ventricle)
I. Head of caudate nucleus
J. Anterior limb of internal capsule
K. Genu of internal capsule
L. Posterior limb of internal capsule
M. Putamen of lentiform nucleus
N. Globus pallidus of lentiform nucleus
O. Thalamus
P. Medial geniculate body
Q. Lateral geniculate body
R. Interthalamic adhesion
S. Third ventricle
T. Superior colliculus (lower tip)

U. Superior (or quadrigeminal) cistern
V. Cerebellum
W. Temporal lobe
X. Tail of caudate nucleus (in roof of *inferior horn of lateral ventricle*)
Y. Hippocampus and its fimbria (in floor of *inferior horn of lateral ventricle*)
Z. From the putamen lateralward: external capsule (white), claustrum (gray), extreme capsule (white), and insula (gray cortex)

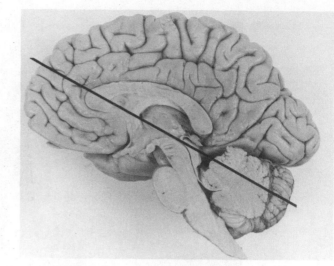

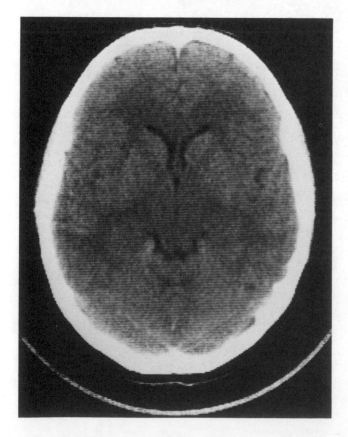

Normal CT scan showing the internal capsule

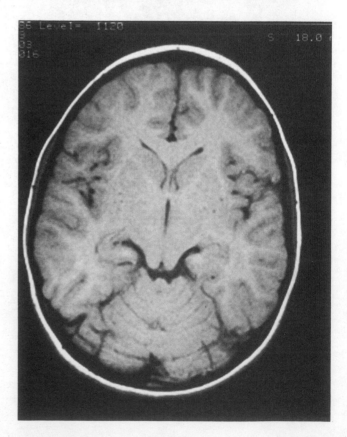

Normal T1-weighted MRI scan

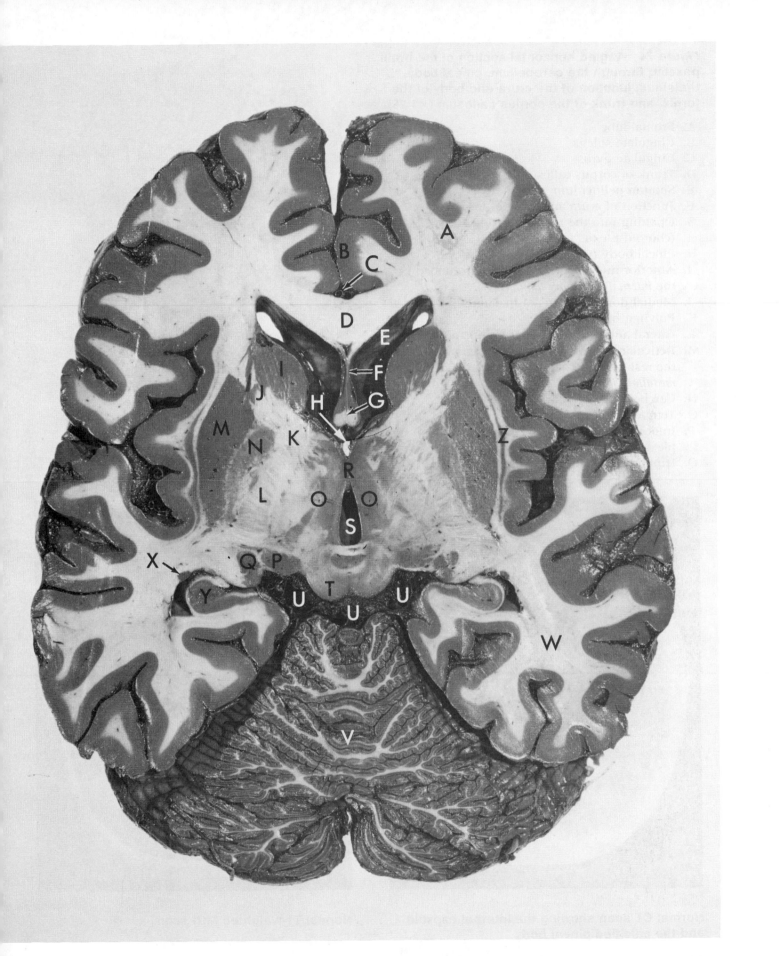

Figure 74 Angled horizontal section of the brain passing through the cerebellum, pineal body, thalamus, junction of the crura and body of the fornix, and trunk of the corpus callosum (×1.25)

A. Frontal lobe
B. Cingulate sulcus
C. Cingulate gyrus
D. Trunk of corpus callosum
E. Septum pellucidum
F. Junction of crura and body of fornix
G. Opening into the roof of third ventricle (choroid plexus is visible)
H. Pineal body (within the *superior cistern*)
I. Anterior nucleus of thalamus (surrounded by the *internal medullary lamina*)
J. Medial dorsal nucleus of thalamus
K. Pulvinar of thalamus
L. Lateral and ventral nuclear groups of thalamus
M. Reticular nucleus of thalamus (separated from the rest of the thalamus by the *external medullary lamina*)
N. Cerebellum
O. Temporal lobe
P. Inferior horn of lateral ventricle (with choroid plexus within it)
Q. Hippocampus and its fimbria

R. Tail of caudate nucleus
S. Posterior limb of internal capsule
T. Genu of internal capsule
U. Anterior limb of internal capsule
V. Anterior horn of lateral ventricle
W. Head of caudate nucleus
X. Putamen
Y. Insula
Z. Lateral sulcus

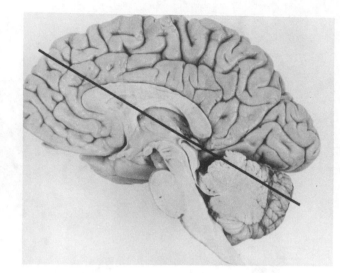

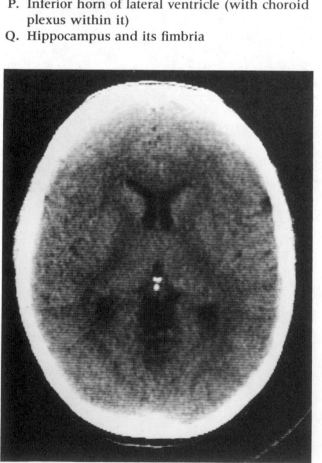

Normal CT scan showing the internal capsule and the calcified pineal body

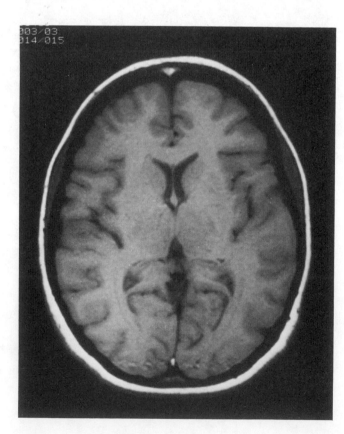

Normal T1-weighted MRI scan

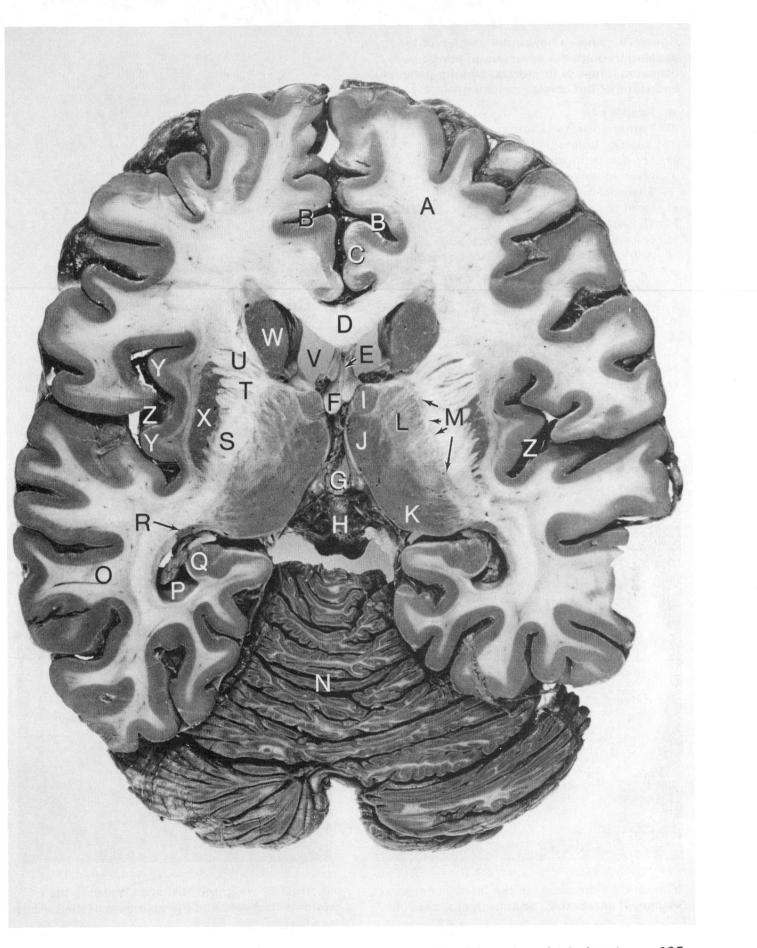

Figure 75 Angled horizontal section of the brain passing through the splenium of the corpus callosum, crura of the fornix, septum pellucidum, and trunk of the corpus callosum (×1.25)

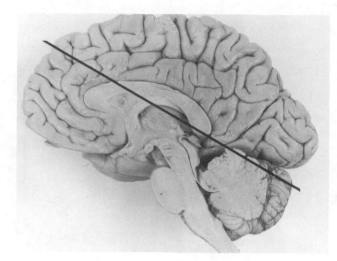

A. Frontal lobe
B. Trunk of corpus callosum
C. Anterior horn of lateral ventricle
D. Septum pellucidum
E. Choroid plexus of lateral ventricle
F. Thalamostriate vein
G. Head of caudate nucleus
H. Thalamus
I. Crus of fornix (cut in two places)
J. Anterior extension of superior cistern within the transverse cerebral fissure (contains the two *internal cerebral veins,* which are difficult to see here)
K. Splenium of corpus callosum
L. Great cerebral vein (within superior cistern)
M. Superior surface of cerebellum
N. Occipital lobe
O. Calcarine sulcus
P. Choroid plexus within inferior horn of lateral ventricle (frequently seen in CT scans at this location)
Q. Tail of caudate nucleus
R. Temporal lobe
S. Corona radiata (just above internal capsule)
T. Lateral sulcus (with several branches of middle cerebral artery within it)

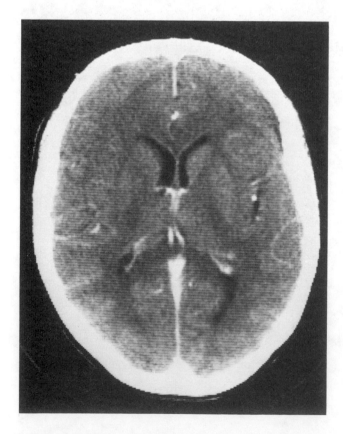

Normal CT scan showing the internal cerebral Vv., great cerebral V., and straight sinus

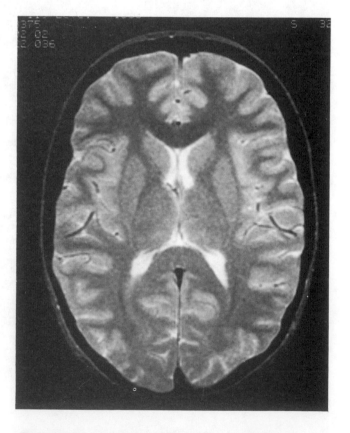

Normal T2-weighted MRI scan showing the internal capsule and the splenium of the corpus callosum

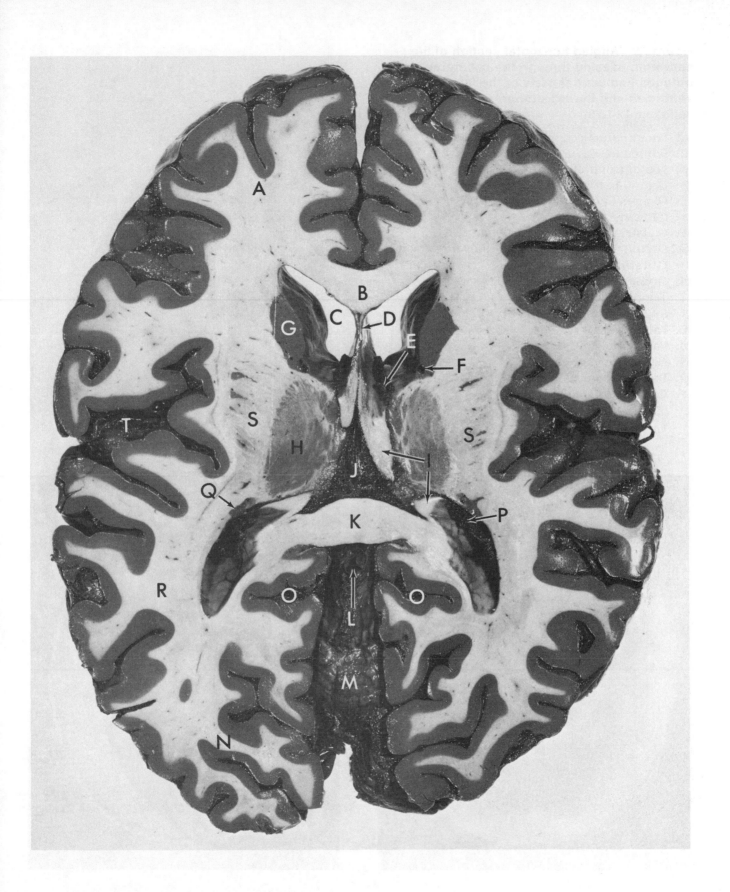

Figure 76 Angled horizontal section of the cerebrum passing through the collateral trigones and central parts of the lateral ventricles and the top of the trunk of the corpus callosum (×1.25)

A. Longitudinal cerebral fissure
B. Frontal lobe
C. Top of trunk of corpus callosum
D. Central part of lateral ventricle
E. Glomus of choroid plexus (frequently seen in CT scans at this location)
F. Collateral trigone of lateral ventricle
G. Occipital forceps of corpus callosum
H. Calcarine sulcus
I. Occipital lobe
J. Temporal lobe
K. Superior temporal sulcus
L. Lateral sulcus
M. Parietal lobe
N. Central sulcus
O. Precentral sulcus
P. Corona radiata

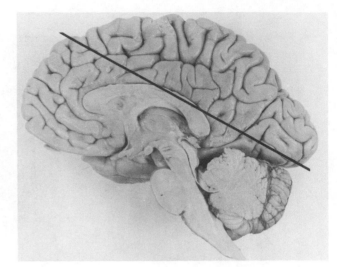

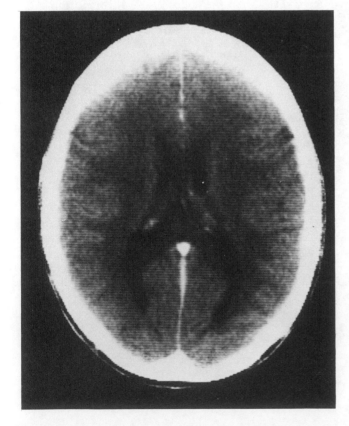

Normal CT scan showing the posterior horns of the lateral ventricles

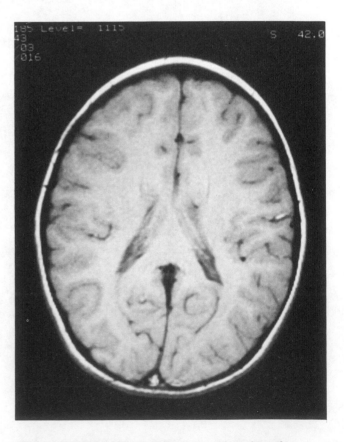

Normal T1-weighted MRI scan showing the glomus of the choroid plexus in the collateral trigone of the lateral ventricle

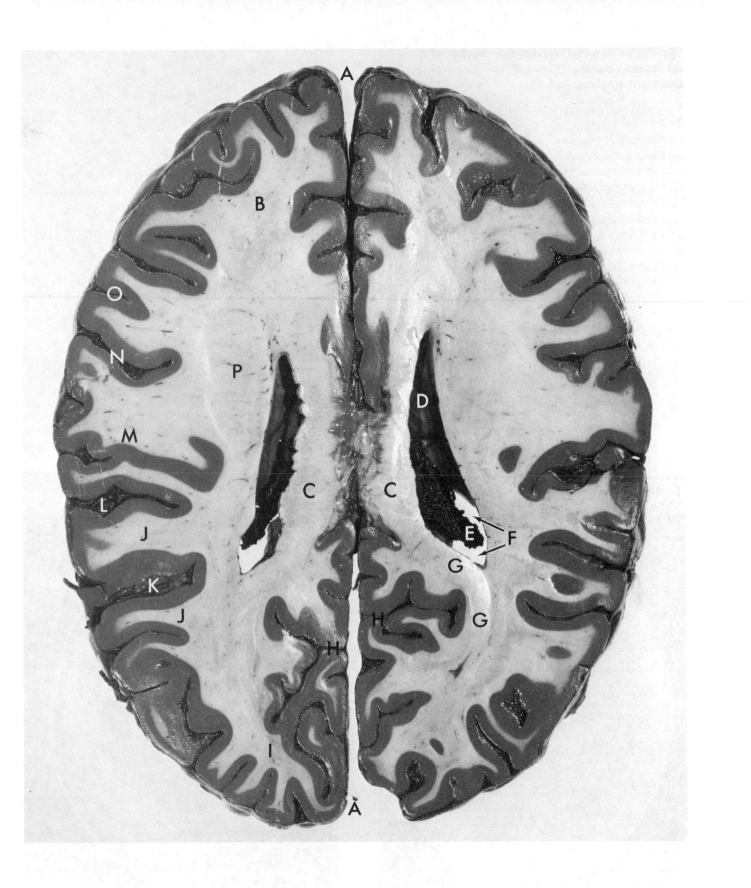

Figure 77 Angled horizontal section of the cerebrum passing through the occipital, parietal, and frontal lobes (×1.25)

A. Longitudinal cerebral fissure
B. Frontal lobe
C. Precentral sulcus
D. Precentral gyrus
E. Central sulcus
F. Postcentral gyrus
G. Postcentral sulcus
H. Parietal lobe
I. Parieto-occipital sulcus
J. Occipital lobe
K. Centrum semiovale

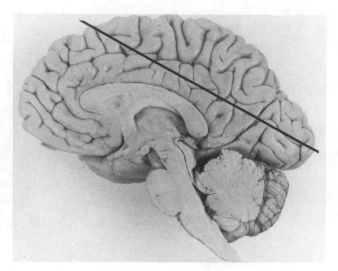

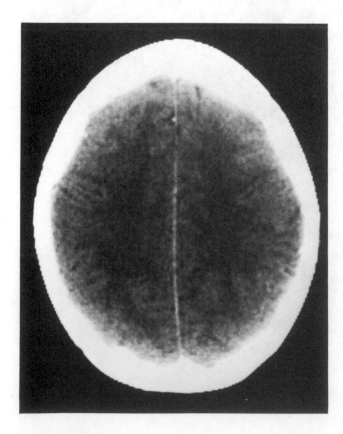

Normal CT scan

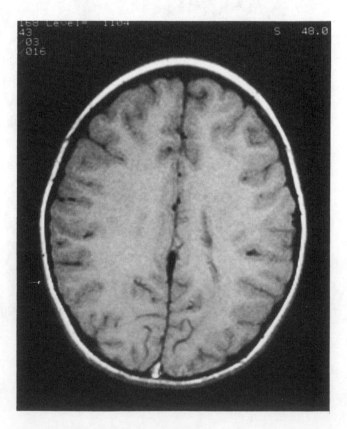

Normal T1-weighted MRI scan

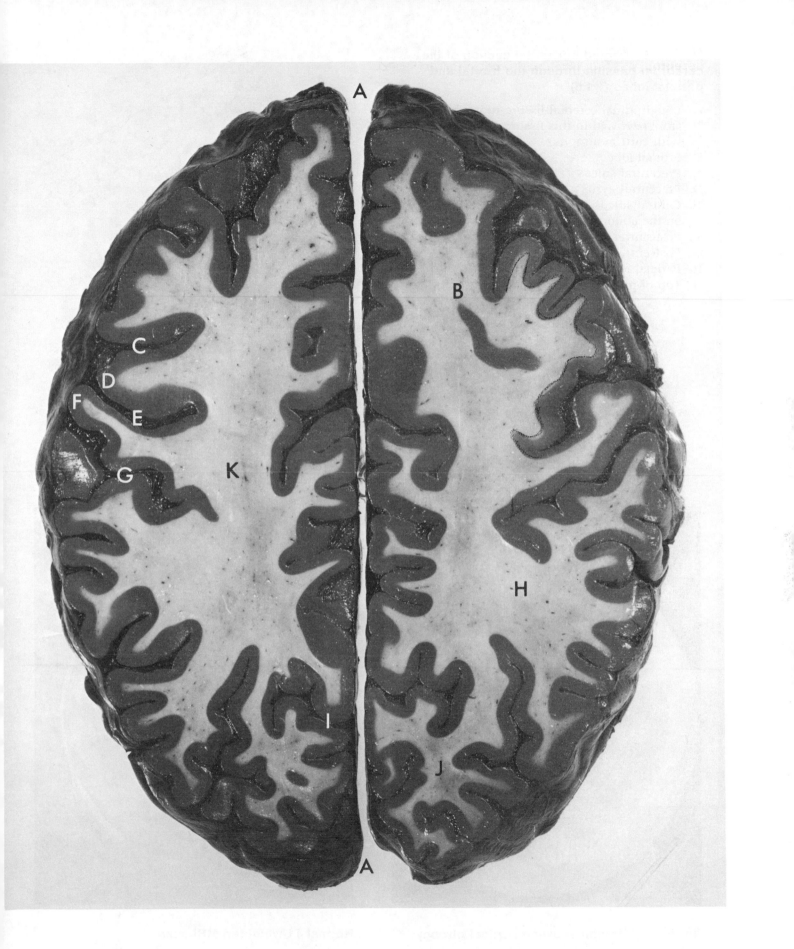

Figure 78 Angled horizontal section of the cerebrum passing through the frontal and parietal lobes (×1.5)

A. Longitudinal cerebral fissure (note the calcified *falx cerebri* within this fissure on the CT scan with cortical atrophy)
B. Frontal lobe
C. Precentral sulcus
D. Precentral gyrus
E. Central sulcus (note the widening of the sulci on the abnormal CT scan with cortical atrophy)
F. Postcentral gyrus
G. Postcentral sulcus
H. Parietal lobe
I. Top of parieto-occipital sulcus

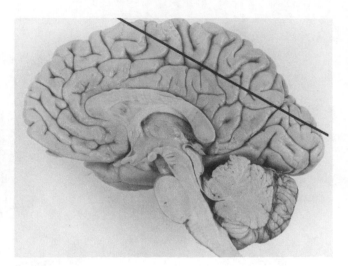

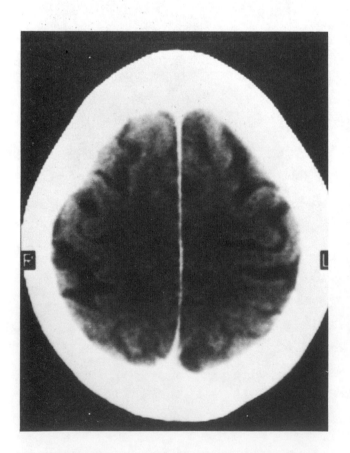

Abnormal CT scan showing cortical atrophy

Normal T1-weighted MRI scan

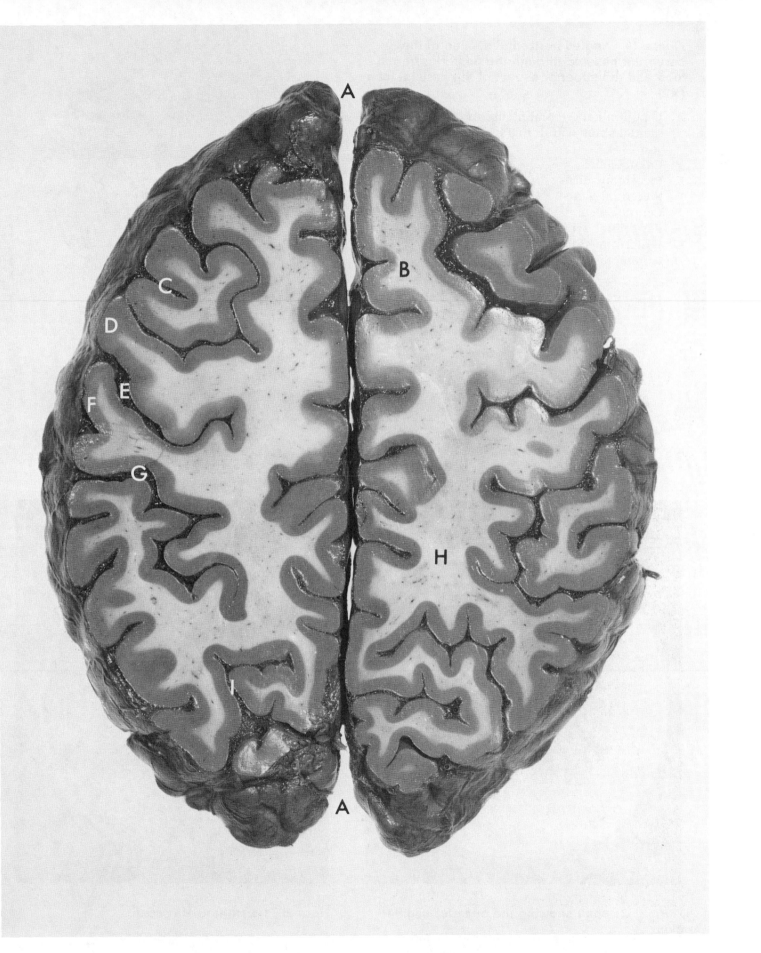

Figure 79 Angled horizontal section of the cerebrum passing through the posterior frontal lobe and the superior aspect of the parietal lobe (×2)

A. Longitudinal cerebral fissure (note the superior sagittal sinus within this fissure on normal CT scan)
B. Frontal lobe
C. Precentral sulcus
D. Precentral gyrus
E. Central sulcus
F. Postcentral gyrus
G. Postcentral sulcus
H. Parietal lobe

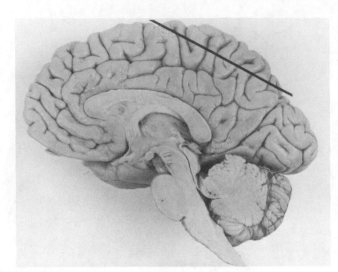

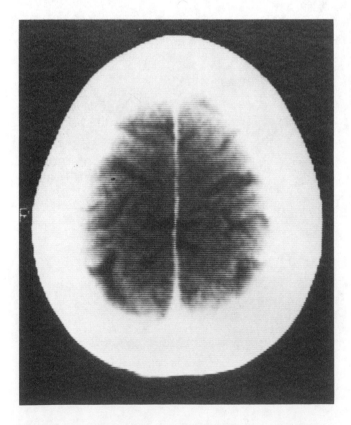

Normal CT scan showing the superior sagittal sinus

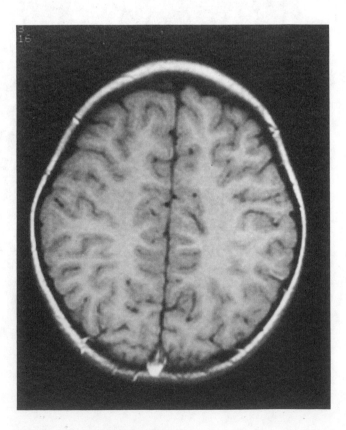

Normal T1-weighted MRI scan

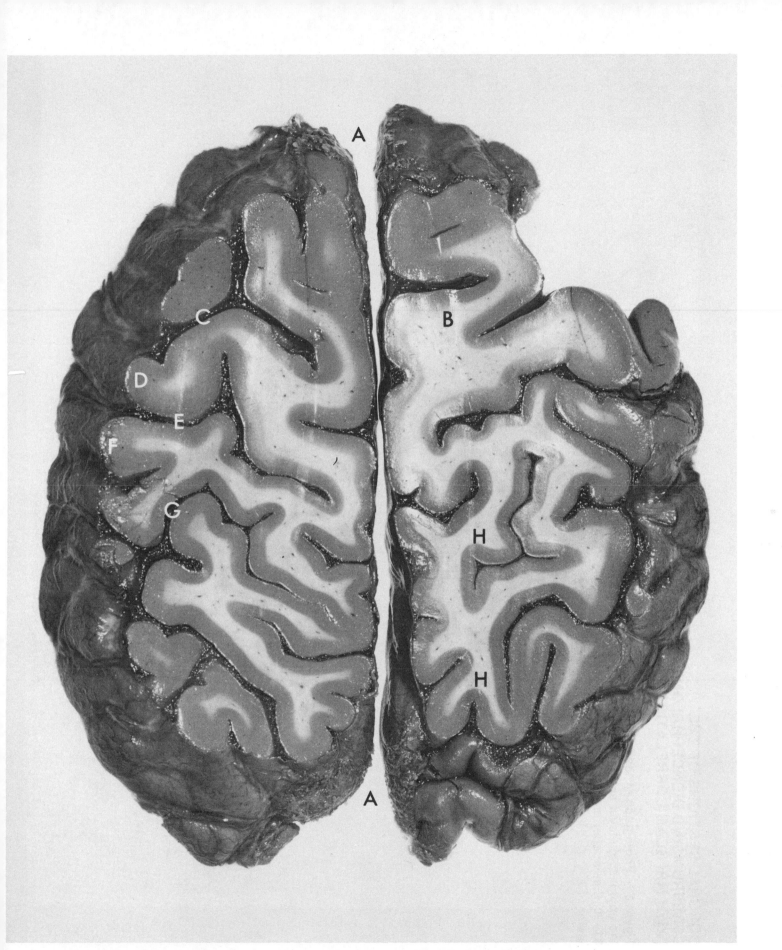

CORONAL SECTIONS OF THE CEREBRUM AND DIENCEPHALON (WITH MRI SCAN CORRELATION)

Figure 80 Photograph of the brain indicating the approximate level and plane of Figures 81–90. (LeMasurier modification of the Mulligan stain)

Atlas of the Brain and Spinal Cord

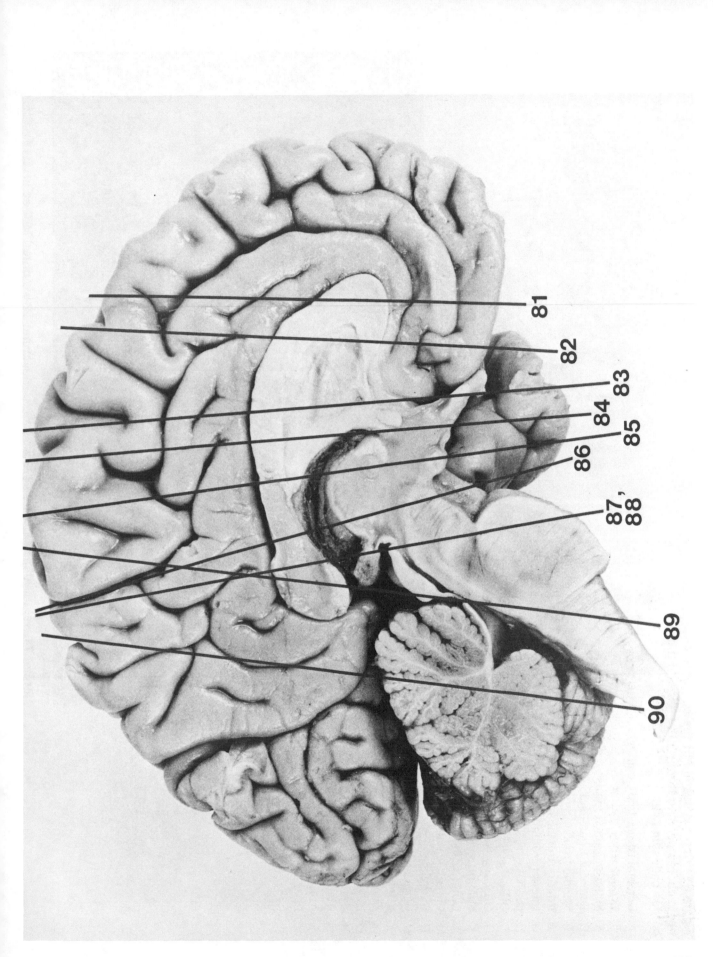

81

82

83

84

85

86

87,
88

89

90

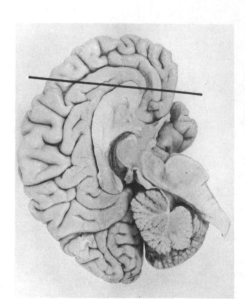

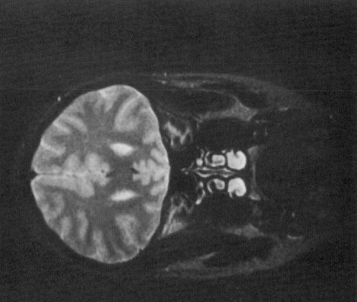

Normal T2-weighted MRI scan

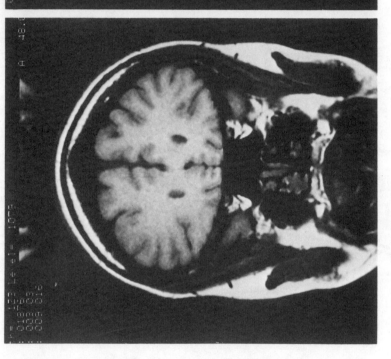

Normal T1-weighted MRI scan

Figure 81 **Coronal section of the cerebral hemispheres passing through the genu of the corpus callosum (×2)**

A. Cerebral cortex (gray matter)
B. Central white matter
C. Superior frontal gyrus
D. Superior frontal sulcus
E. Middle frontal gyrus
F. Inferior frontal sulcus
G. Inferior frontal gyrus
H. Orbital gyri
I. Orbital sulci
J. Olfactory sulcus
K. Straight gyrus (gyrus rectus)
L. Longitudinal cerebral fissure
M. Cingulate sulcus
N. Cingulate gyrus
O. Genu of corpus callosum
P. Anterior horn of right lateral ventricle
Q. Head of caudate nucleus
R. Anterior cerebral arteries (two places)
S. Arachnoid (spans the sulcus)
T. Pia mater (dips into the sulcus)

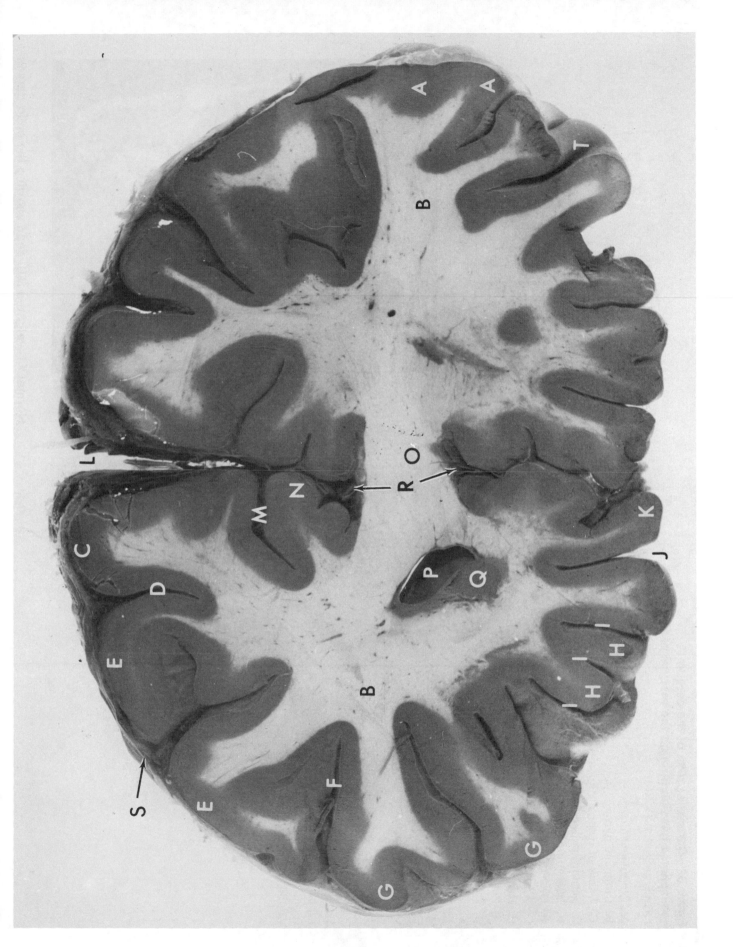

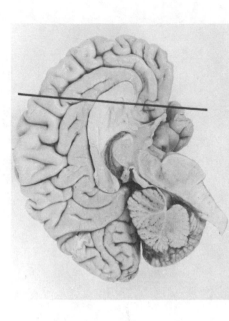

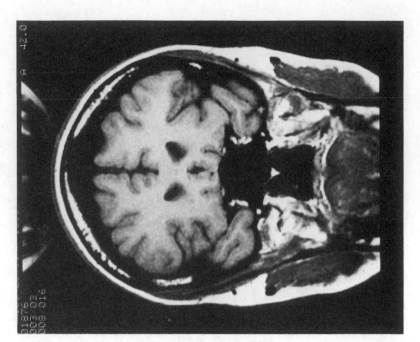

Normal T1-weighted MRI scan showing the optic nerves

Figure 82 **Coronal section of the cerebral hemispheres passing through the rostrum of the corpus callosum (×1.5)**

A. Cingulate sulcus
B. Cingulate gyrus
C. Trunk of corpus callosum
D. Septum pellucidum
E. Rostrum of corpus callosum
F. Olfactory tract (in olfactory sulcus)
G. Anterior horn of lateral ventricle
H. Head of caudate nucleus
I. Putamen (of lentiform nucleus)
J. External capsule
K. Claustrum
L. Extreme capsule
M. Middle cerebral artery (in lateral sulcus)
N. Temporal lobe
O. Arachnoid (spans the sulci)

Can you locate:

Longitudinal cerebral fissure
Anterior cerebral arteries
Superior, middle, and inferior frontal gyri
Superior and inferior frontal sulci
Medial frontal gyrus

150   *Atlas of the Brain and Spinal Cord*

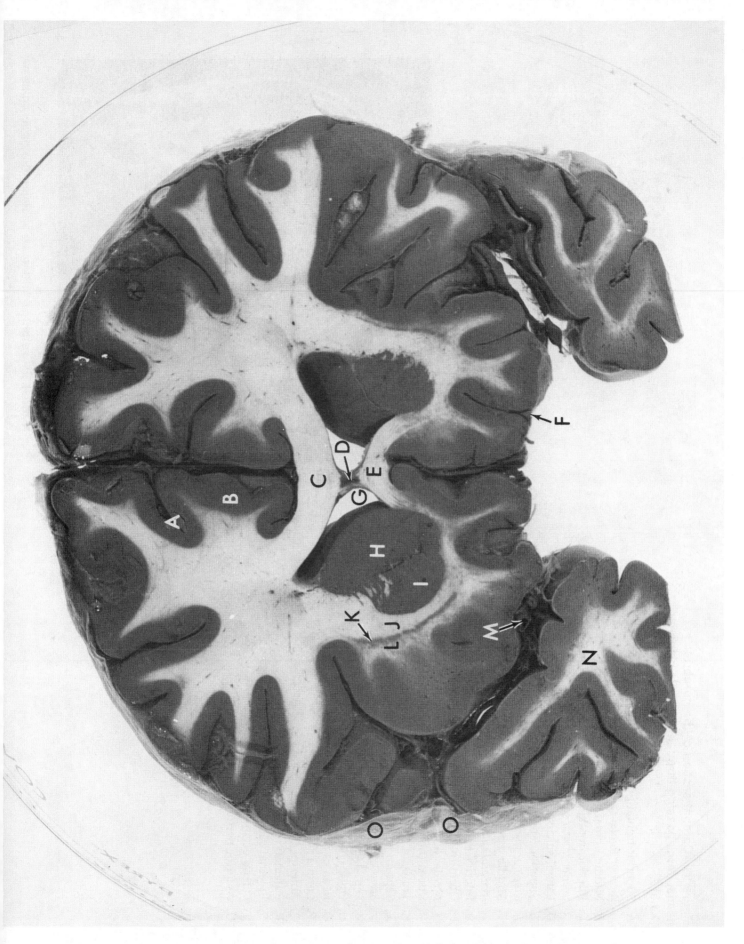

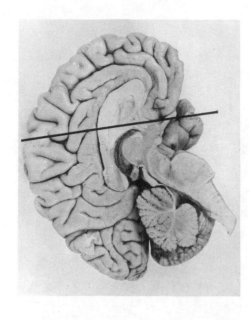

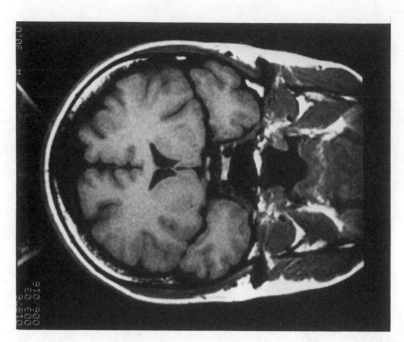

Normal T1-weighted MRI scan showing the optic chiasma

Figure 83 **Coronal section of the cerebral hemispheres passing through the optic chiasma (×1.5)**

A. Superior frontal gyrus (bounded inferiorly by *superior frontal sulcus*)
B. Middle frontal gyrus
C. Inferior frontal gyrus (bounded superiorly by *inferior frontal sulcus*)
D. Lateral sulcus
E. Superior temporal gyrus (bounded by *superior temporal sulcus* inferiorly)
F. Middle temporal gyrus (bounded by *inferior temporal sulcus* inferiorly)
G. Inferior temporal gyrus
H. Occipitotemporal sulcus
I. Medial occipitotemporal gyrus
J. Uncus (bounded laterally by *rhinal sulcus*)
K. Trunk of corpus callosum
L. Septum pellucidum (separating the *anterior horns of left and right lateral ventricles*)
M. Septal area — paraterminal gyrus
N. Optic chiasma
O. Head of caudate nucleus
P. Corona radiata
Q. Anterior limb of internal capsule
R. Putamen of lentiform nucleus
S. External capsule
T. Lateral occipitotemporal gyrus
U. Anterior perforated substance

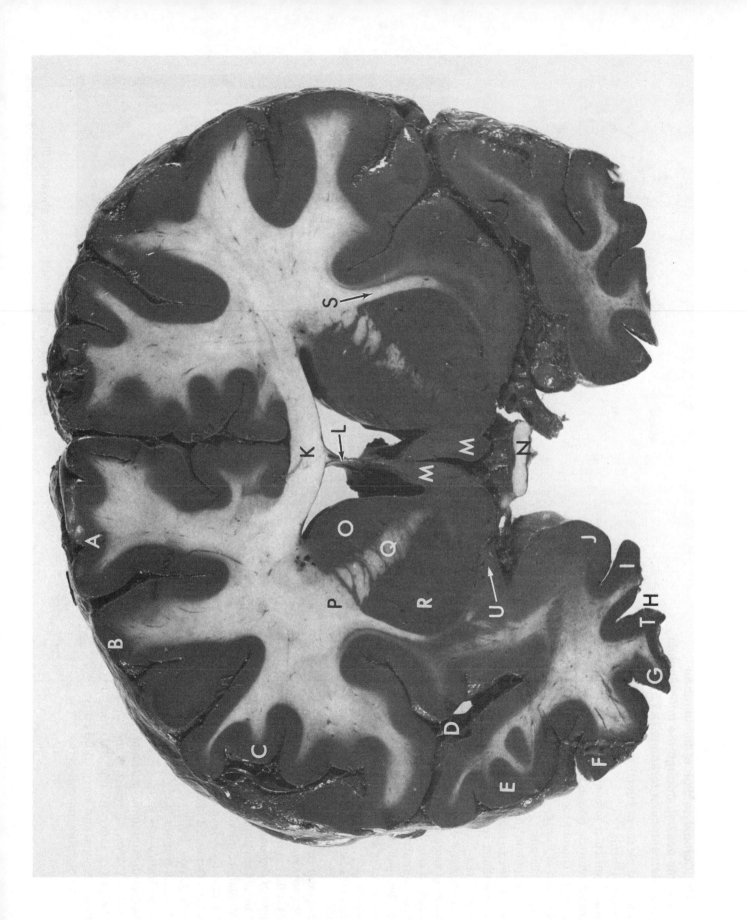

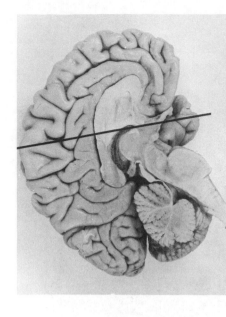

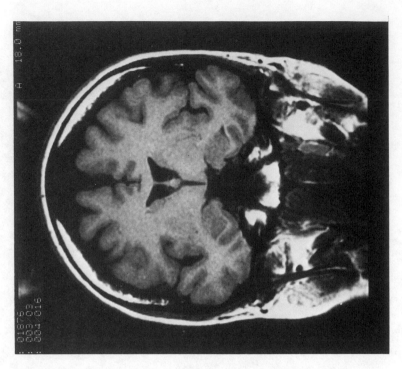

Normal T1-weighted MRI scan showing the interventricular foramina and the amygdaloid bodies

Figure 84 **Coronal section of the cerebral hemispheres passing through the infundibulum and the interventricular foramina (×1.5)**

A. Choroid plexus of lateral ventricle
B. Body of fornix
C. Interventricular foramen
D. Third ventricle (locate the hypothalamic sulcus and the choroid plexus)
E. Column of fornix
F. Hypothalamus
G. Infundibulum (note that the cavity of the third ventricle extends into the infundibulum as the infundibular recess)
H. Optic tract
I. Anterior end of thalamus
J. Body of caudate nucleus
K. Internal capsule (near *genu*)
L. Corona radiata
M. Globus pallidus of lentiform nucleus
N. Putamen of lentiform nucleus
O. Insula
P. Lateral sulcus (with middle cerebral artery in it)
Q. Superior temporal gyrus (bounded inferiorly by *superior temporal sulcus*)
R. Middle temporal gyrus (bounded inferiorly by *inferior temporal sulcus*)
S. Inferior temporal gyrus
T. Medial occipitotemporal gyrus (bounded laterally by *occipitotemporal sulcus*)
U. Uncus (bounded laterally by *rhinal sulcus*)
V. Amygdaloid body
W. Anterior commissure
X. Ansa lenticularis
Y. Substantia innominata (contains the *basal nucleus* [Meynert], which is the source of cholinergic innervation of the cerebral cortex, hippocampus, and amygdaloid body)
Z. Lateral occipitotemporal gyrus

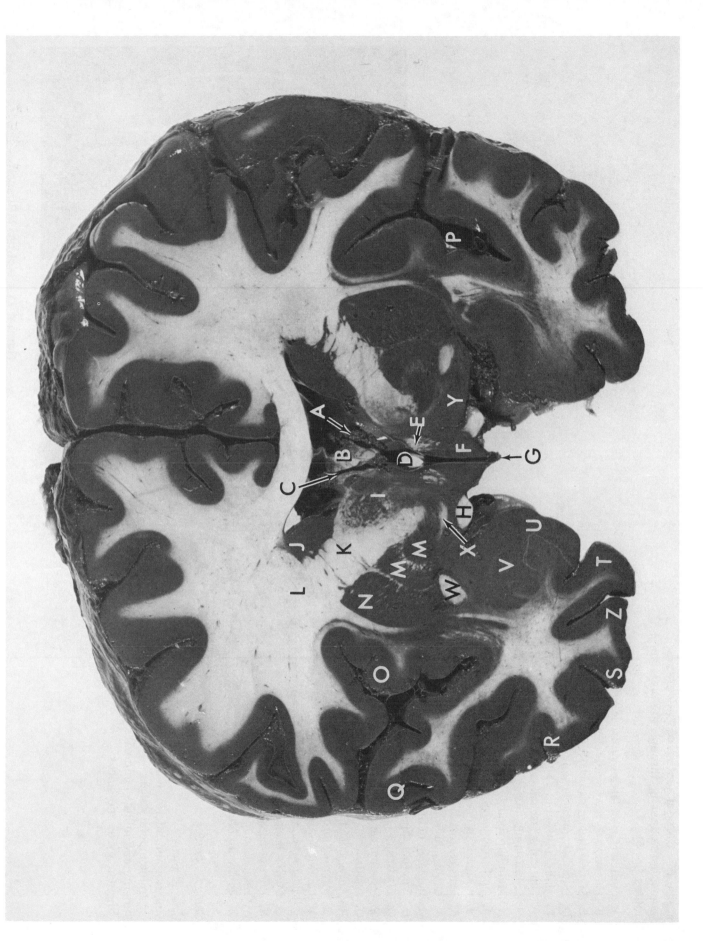

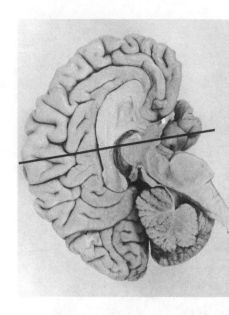

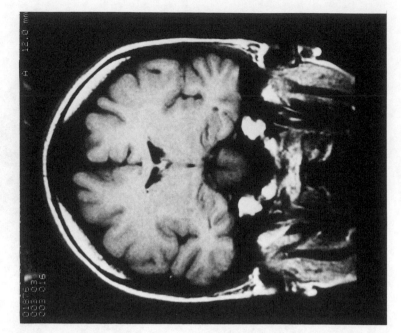

Normal T1-weighted MRI scan

Figure 85 **Coronal section of the cerebral hemispheres passing through the mamillary bodies (×1.5)**

A. Central part of lateral ventricle
B. Lateral thalamic nuclei
C. Medial thalamic nuclei
D. Interthalamic adhesion
E. Mamillothalamic tract
F. Lenticular fasciculus
G. Subthalamic nucleus
H. Mamillary body
I. Optic tract
J. Posterior limb of internal capsule
K. Crus cerebri of cerebral peduncle
L. Globus pallidus of lentiform nucleus
M. Putamen of lentiform nucleus
N. External capsule
O. Claustrum
P. Extreme capsule
Q. Insula
R. Amygdaloid body
S. Inferior horn of lateral ventricle
T. Parahippocampal gyrus (bounded laterally by *collateral sulcus*)
U. Medial occipitotemporal gyrus
V. Inferior temporal gyrus
W. Lateral occipitotemporal gyrus
X. Paracentral lobule

Can you locate:

Lateral sulcus
Superior and inferior temporal sulci
Occipitotemporal sulcus
Superior and middle temporal gyri
Cingulate gyrus and sulcus

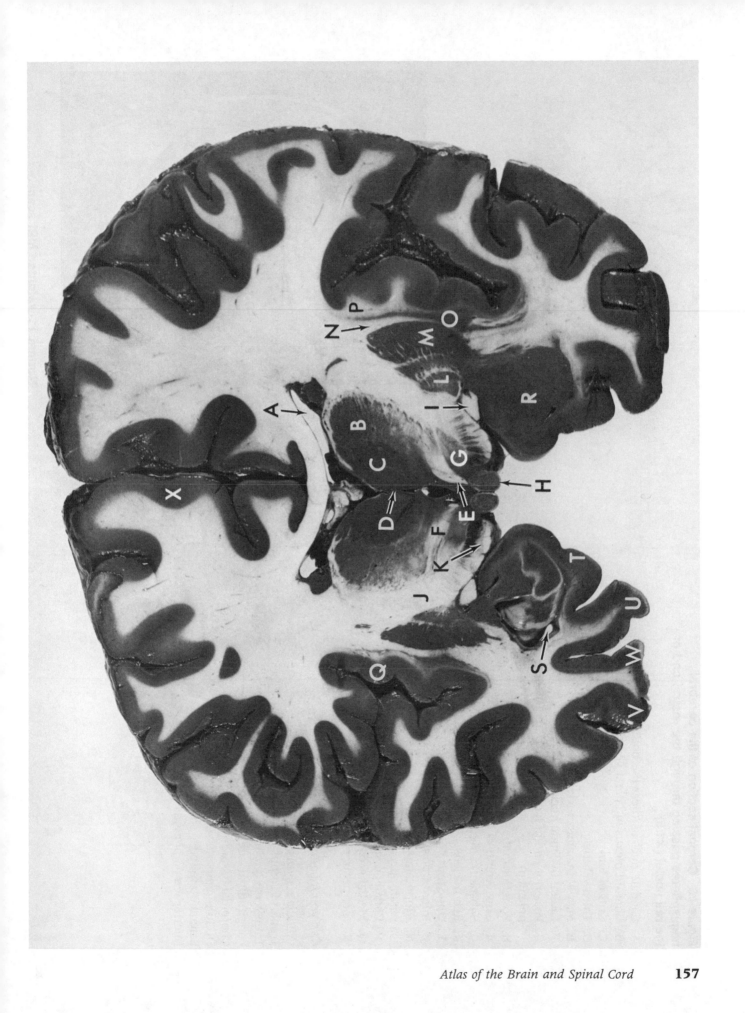

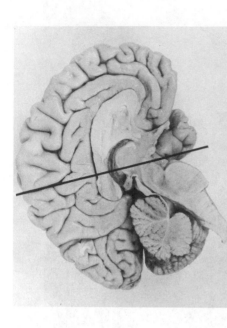

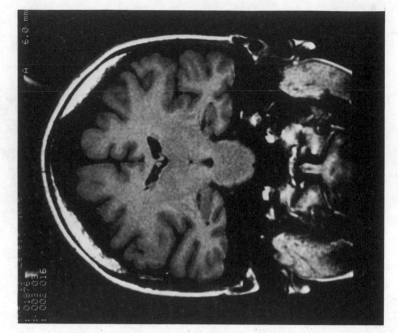

Normal T1-weighted MRI scan

Figure 86 **Coronal section of the cerebral hemispheres passing through the rostral end of the red nuclei (×1.5)**

A. Caudate nucleus (near the body–tail juncture)
B. Choroid plexus of lateral ventricle
C. Crus of fornix
D. Third ventricle
E. Medial thalamic nuclei
F. Lateral thalamic nuclei
G. Posterior end of lentiform nucleus (mostly putamen)
H. Posterior limb of internal capsule
I. Crus cerebri of cerebral peduncle
J. Substantia nigra of cerebral peduncle
K. Red nucleus
L. Optic tract
M. Inferior horn of lateral ventricle
N. Hippocampus
O. Parahippocampal gyrus
P. Collateral sulcus
Q. Medial occipitotemporal gyrus
R. Interpeduncular fossa

Can you locate:

Cingulate gyrus and sulcus
Trunk of corpus callosum
Transverse cerebral fissure
Longitudinal cerebral fissure
Choroidal fissure
Occipitotemporal sulcus
Lateral occipitotemporal gyrus
Inferior temporal gyrus

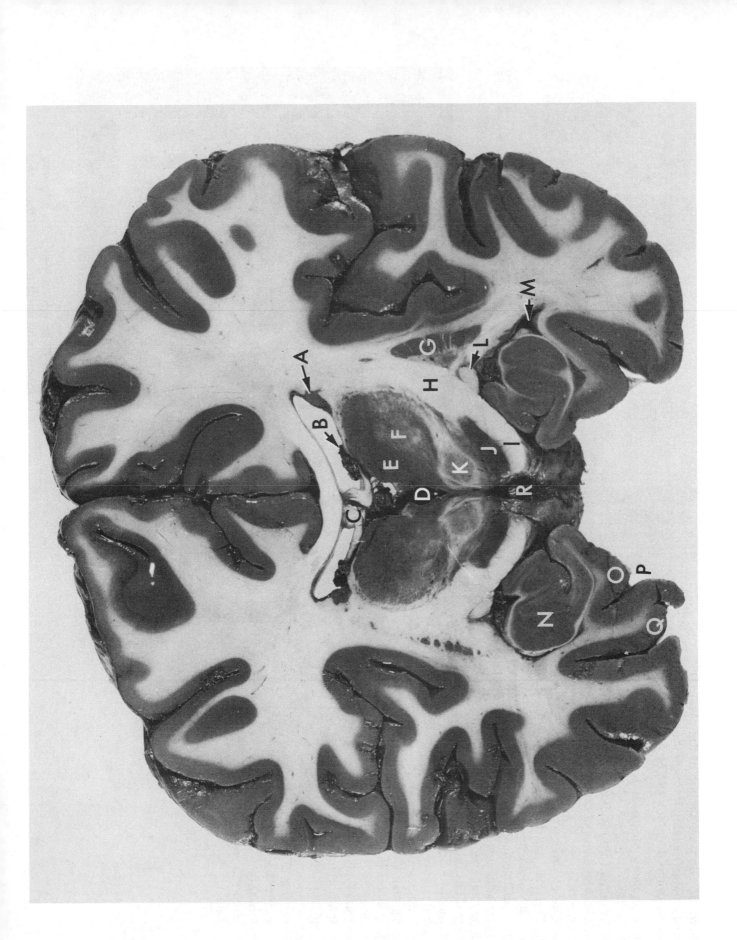

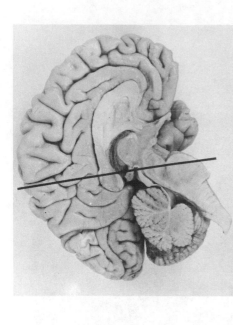

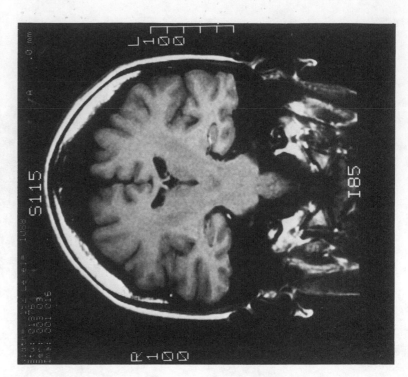

Normal T1-weighted MRI scan showing the hippocampus and the crus of the fornix

Figure 87 **Coronal section of the cerebral hemispheres passing through the geniculate bodies of the thalamus (×1.5)**

A. Cingulate gyrus (bounded above by *cingulate sulcus*)
B. Trunk of corpus callosum
C. Choroid plexus of central part of lateral ventricle
D. Crus of fornix
E. Thalamus (pulvinar)
F. Lateral geniculate body
G. Medial geniculate body
H. Pretectal area
I. Central gray substance of midbrain (hole in the middle of this is the *cerebral aqueduct*)
J. Medial longitudinal fasciculus
K. Superior cerebellar peduncle (soon to enter the red nucleus rostrally)
L. Substantia nigra of cerebral peduncle
M. Crus cerebri of cerebral peduncle
N. Pons
O. Tail of caudate nucleus (two places)
P. Inferior horn of lateral ventricle (with choroid plexus)
Q. Hippocampus
R. Fimbria of hippocampus (two places)
S. Parahippocampal gyrus
T. Pineal body (in the anterior extension of the *superior cistern* within the *transverse cerebral fissure*)

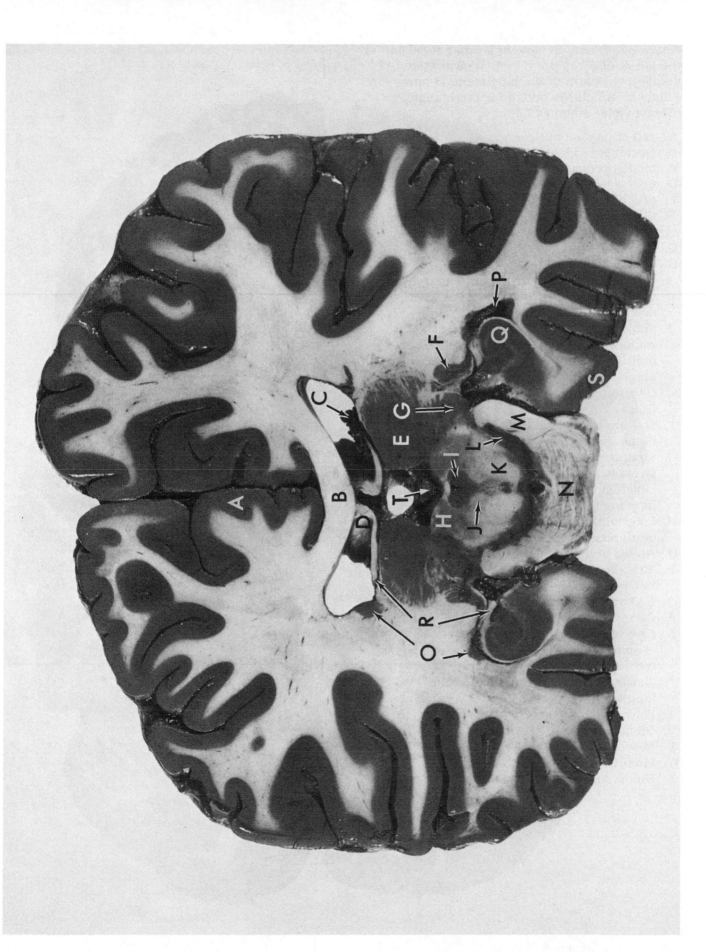

Figure 88 Close-up view of a coronal section of the left medial temporal lobe showing the detailed structure of the hippocampal formation. Adjacent structures added for orientation. (Cresyl violet stain) (×9.5)

A. Tail of caudate nucleus
B. Lateral geniculate body
C. Medial geniculate body
D. Crus cerebri of midbrain
E. Choroidal fissure
F. Choroid plexus of inferior horn of lateral ventricle
G. Inferior horn of lateral ventricle
H. Collateral sulcus
I. Parahippocampal gyrus (entorhinal cortex, which represents transitional six-layered neocortex)
J. Subiculum (as well as *presubiculum* and *parasubiculum*, which represent *paleocortex* in transition to the three-layered *archicortex* of the hippocampus)
K. CA1 sector of hippocampus (pyramidal cell layer)
L. Stratum lacunosum and stratum moleculare of hippocampus
M. Stratum radiatum of hippocampus [these three layers (strata radiatum, lacunosum, and moleculare) make up the *molecular layer* of the hippocampus]
N. Polymorphic layer (stratum oriens) and alveus of hippocampus
O. Alveus of hippocampus
P. Stratum oriens (polymorphic layer) of hippocampus
Q. CA2 sector of hippocampus (pyramidal layer)
R. CA3 sector of hippocampus (pyramidal layer)
S. CA4 sector of hippocampus (pyramidal layer) — some authors believe this zone should be considered part of the *polymorphic layer of the dentate gyrus* rather than a part of the hippocampus
T. Polymorphic layer of dentate gyrus
U. Granular (granule cell) layer of dentate gyrus
V. Molecular layer of dentate gyrus
W. Fimbria of hippocampus
X. Hippocampal sulcus

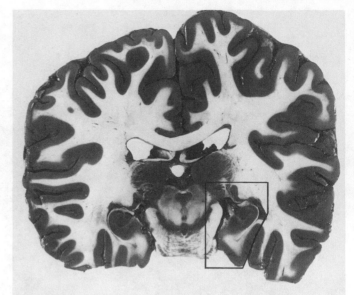

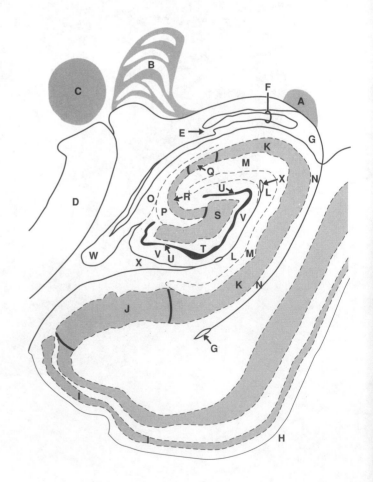

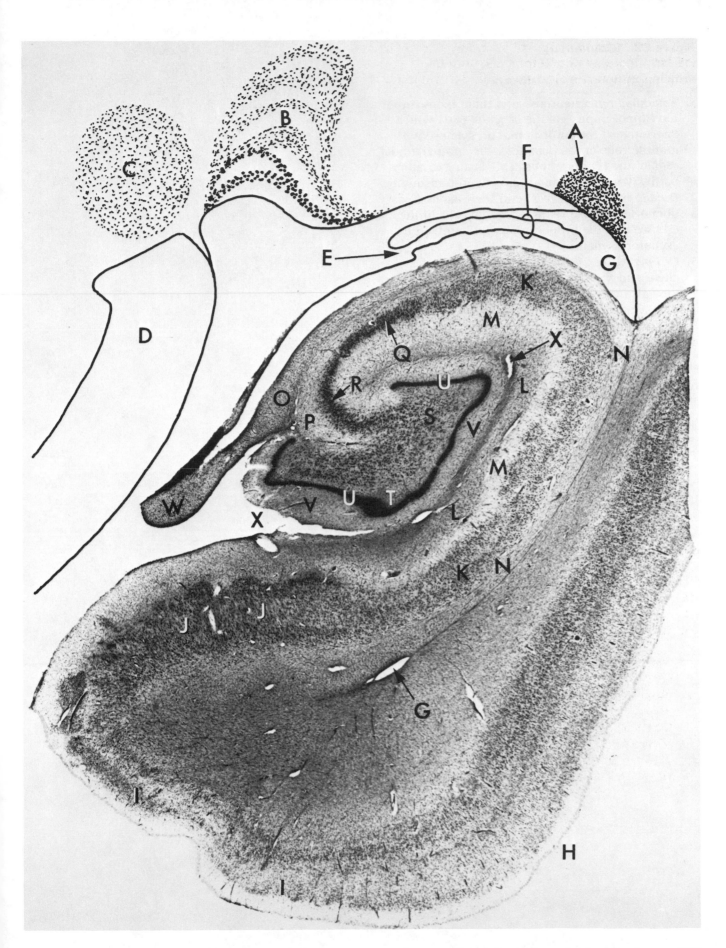

Figure 88 *(Continued)*

Principal Hippocampal Pathways

1. *Entorhinal cortex* neurons send their axons into the hippocampus via the *perforant path,* which "perforates" the subiculum, and synapse with granule cells of the dentate gyrus and pyramidal cells of the hippocampus. This is an excitatory pathway using glutamate as a neurotransmitter.

2. *Dentate gyrus granule cells* send their axons (mossy fibers) to synapse with pyramidal cells in the *CA3 sector* of the hippocampus (glutaminergic excitatory synapse).

3. *CA3 pyramidal cells* send their axons into the *alveus* and *fimbria* of the hippocampus. However, they also give off *recurrent (Schaffer) collaterals* that synapse with CA1 pyramidal cells (glutaminergic excitatory synapse).

4. *CA1 pyramidal cells* send their axons into the *alveus* and then *fimbria* of the hippocampus as another output of the hippocampus. However, collaterals of these axons synapse with neurons of the subiculum.

5. Neurons of the *subiculum* form the major output of the hippocampus by sending their axons into the alveus and then fimbria of the hippocampus to enter the fornix and distribute to the mamillary bodies, septal region, and hypothalamus. Ultimately, these projections reach the thalamus and cerebral cortex (especially cingulate gyrus).

6. Neurons of the subiculum also project back to the *entorhinal cortex,* which has connections with cortical association areas.

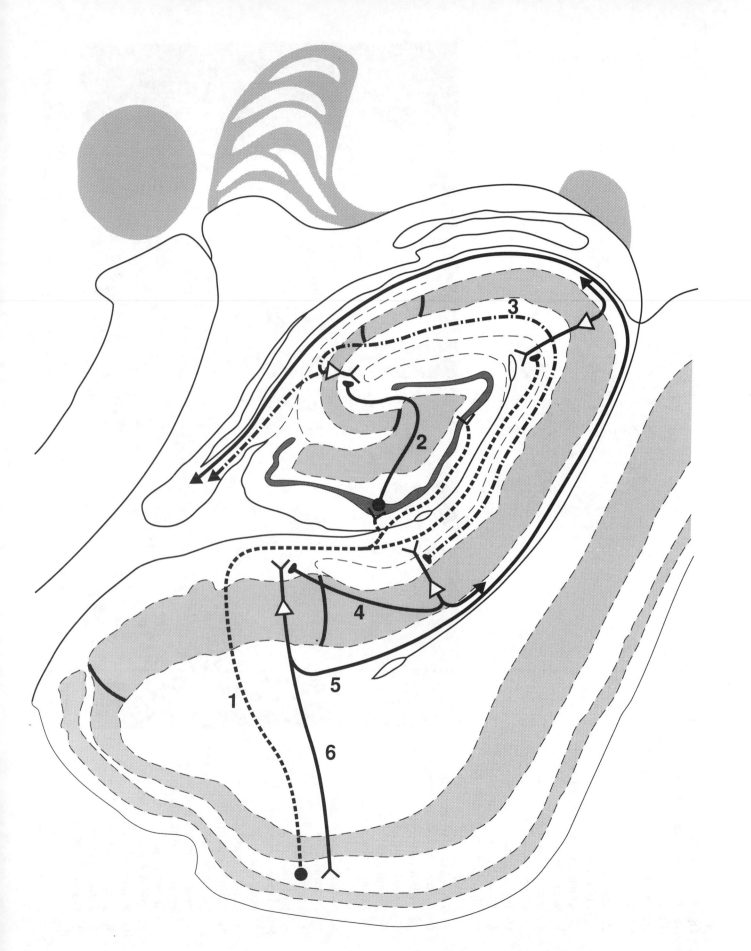

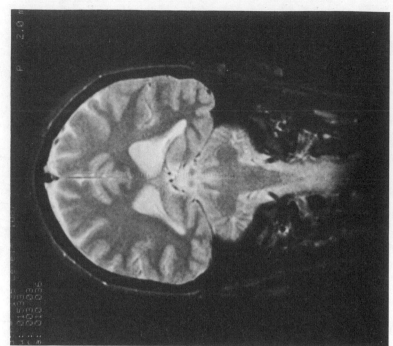

Normal T2-weighted MRI scan showing the collateral trigone and inferior horn of the lateral ventricle

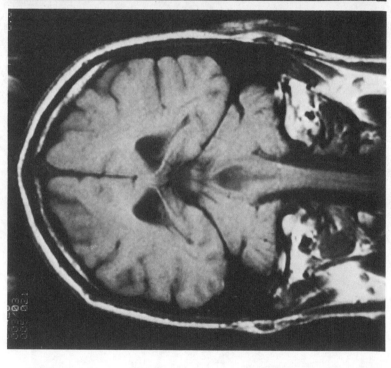

Normal T1-weighted MRI scan showing the collateral trigone and inferior horn of the lateral ventricle

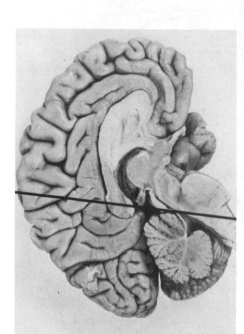

Figure 89 **Coronal section of the cerebral hemispheres passing through the splenium of the corpus callosum and the collateral trigones and inferior horns of the lateral ventricles (×1.25)**

A. Splenium of corpus callosum
B. Collateral trigone of lateral ventricle
C. Inferior horn of lateral ventricle
D. Hippocampus
E. Transition from fimbria of hippocampus to crus of fornix
F. Tail of caudate nucleus
G. Glomus of choroid plexus within collateral trigone of lateral ventricle
H. Pulvinar of thalamus
I. Superior cistern
J. Inferior colliculus
K. Superior cerebellar peduncle
L. Middle cerebellar peduncle
M. Inferior cerebellar peduncle
N. Fourth ventricle
O. Medial longitudinal fasciculus (MLF) (superior to arrow head) and medial lemniscus (inferior to arrow head)
P. Inferior olivary nucleus
Q. Pyramidal tract
R. Cerebellar hemisphere
S. Temporal lobe
T. Parietal lobe

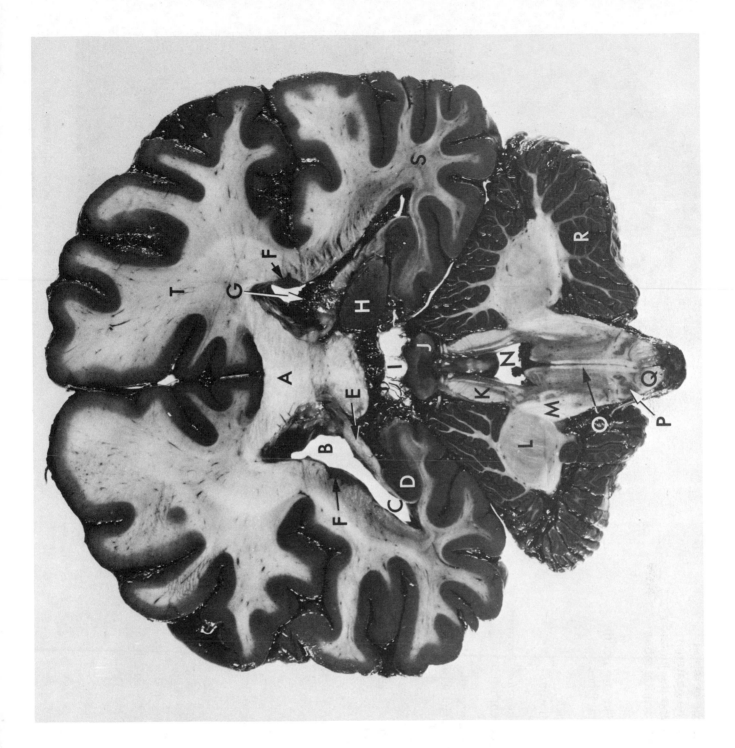

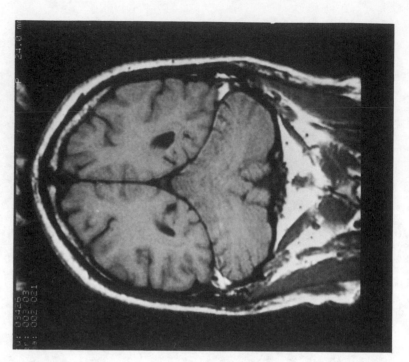

Normal T1-weighted MRI scan showing the posterior horn of the lateral ventricle

Figure 90 **Coronal section of the cerebral hemispheres passing through the posterior horns of the lateral ventricles and the junction of the temporal, parietal, and occipital lobes (×2)**

A. Central white matter near the junction of the parietal, occipital, and temporal lobes
B. Tapetum of corpus callosum
C. Posterior horn of lateral ventricle
D. Occipital forceps of corpus callosum
E. Position of optic radiations
F. Calcarine sulcus (producing the *calcar avis* of the posterior horn of the lateral ventricle)
G. Lingual gyrus
H. Collateral sulcus (which produces the *collateral eminence* in the floor of the posterior and inferior horns of the ventricle)
I. Medial occipitotemporal gyrus
J. Occipitotemporal sulcus
K. Lateral occipitotemporal gyrus
L. Longitudinal cerebral fissure

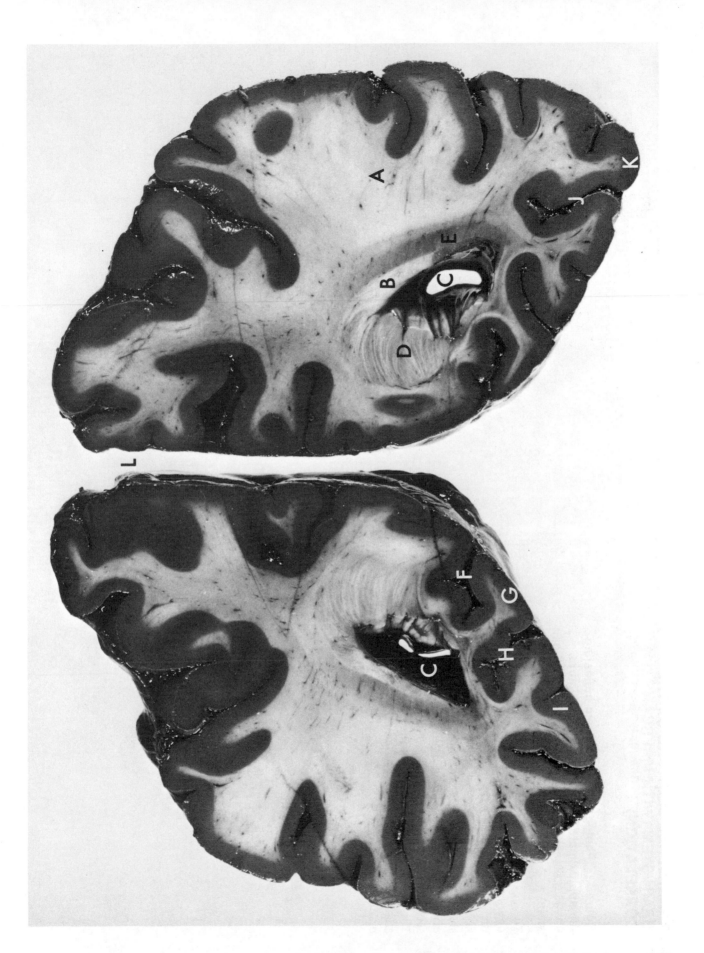

TRANSVERSE SECTIONS OF THE BRAIN STEM (WITH MRI SCAN CORRELATION)

Figure 91 **Photograph of the brain indicating the approximate level and plane of Figures 92–96 (LeMasurier modification of the Mulligan stain)**

The next five sections of the brain stem are oriented as they are viewed in MRI scans, rather than the way they are commonly presented in neuroanatomical texts and atlases. The student should become familiar with both methods of orientation, and it is hoped that presenting the sections in both ways will facilitate that process. The sections in the Weigert-stained brain stem atlas (Figures 104–117) are oriented in the usual manner.

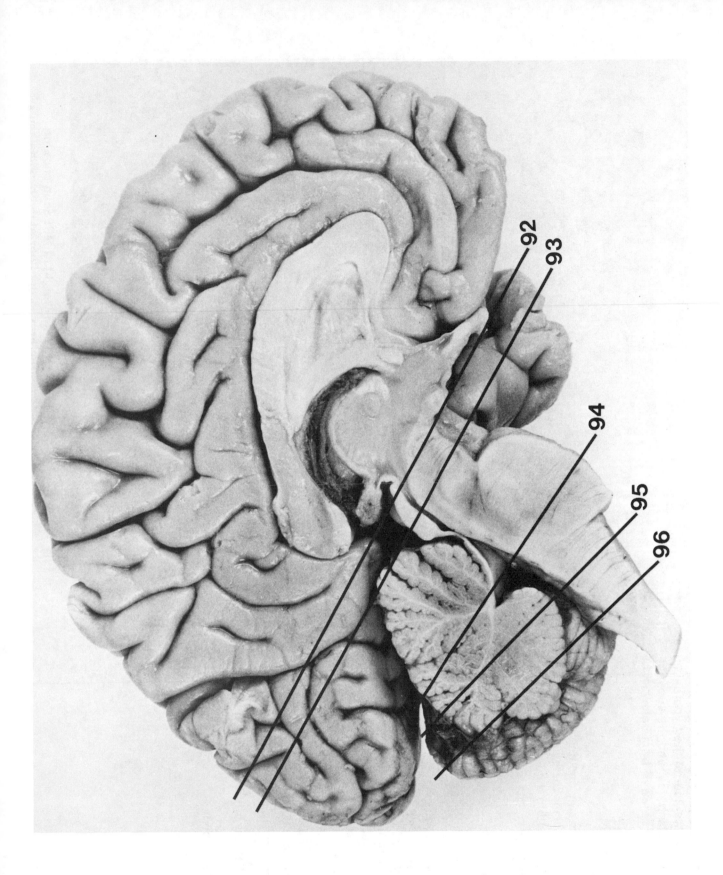

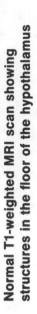

Normal T1-weighted MRI scan showing structures in the floor of the hypothalamus

Figure 92 **Transverse section of the midbrain passing through the floor of the hypothalamus, the cerebral hemispheres, and the superior colliculi. Section is viewed from below (×1.5)**

A. Optic nerve (II)
B. Optic chiasma
C. Optic tract
D. Tuber cinereum (the opening directly behind the optic chiasma is the *infundibular recess of the third ventricle within the infundibulum*)
E. Mamillary body
F. Crus cerebri
G. Substantia nigra
H. Red nucleus
I. Central gray substance (the opening in the middle of this is the *cerebral aqueduct*)
J. Superior colliculus
K. Medial geniculate body
L. Optic tract
M. Lateral geniculate body
N. Pulvinar of thalamus
O. Splenium of corpus callosum
P. Parieto-occipital sulcus
Q. Occipital forceps of corpus callosum
R. Glomus of choroid plexus within collateral trigone of lateral ventricle
S. Optic radiations
T. Hippocampus
U. Choroid plexus within inferior horn of lateral ventricle
V. Amygdaloid body
W. Uncus

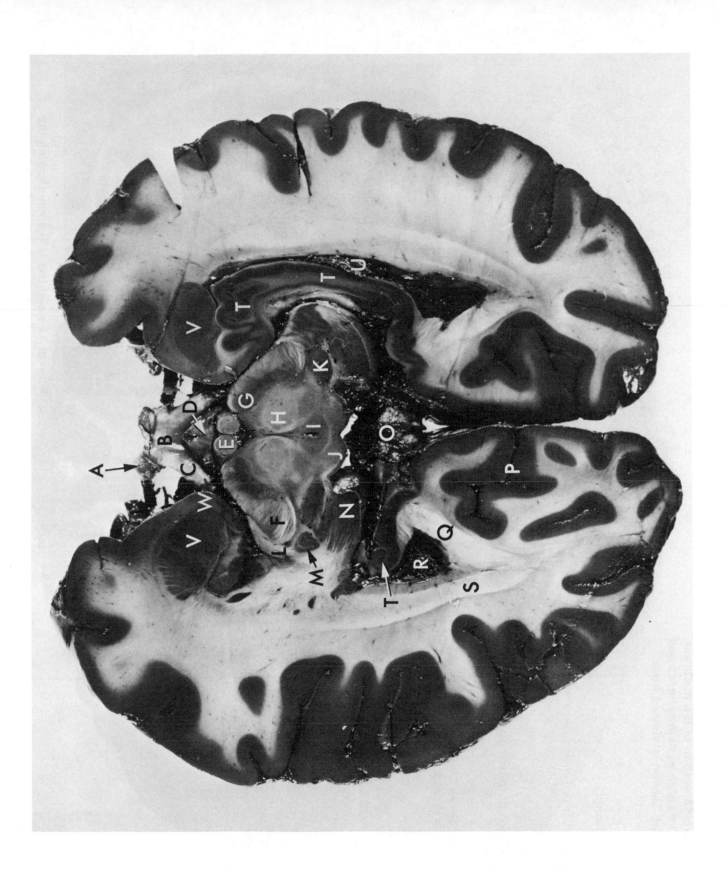

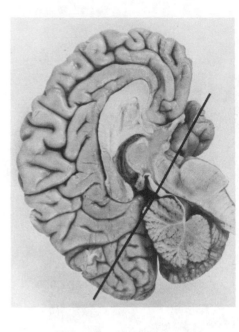

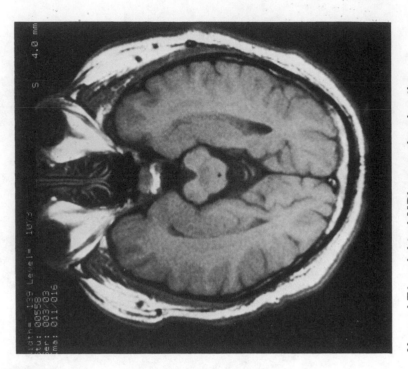

Normal T1-weighted MRI scan showing the inferior horn of the lateral ventricle

Figure 93 **Transverse section of the midbrain passing through the cerebral hemispheres and the inferior colliculi. Section is viewed from below (×1.5)**

A. Uncus
B. Inferior tip of mamillary body
C. Crus cerebri
D. Superior cerebellar peduncle (just above its decussation)
E. Cerebral aqueduct
F. Inferior colliculus
G. Calcarine sulcus (cut in two places)
H. Optic radiations
I. Posterior horn of lateral ventricle
J. Inferior horn of lateral ventricle
K. Hippocampus (sectioned along its long axis)

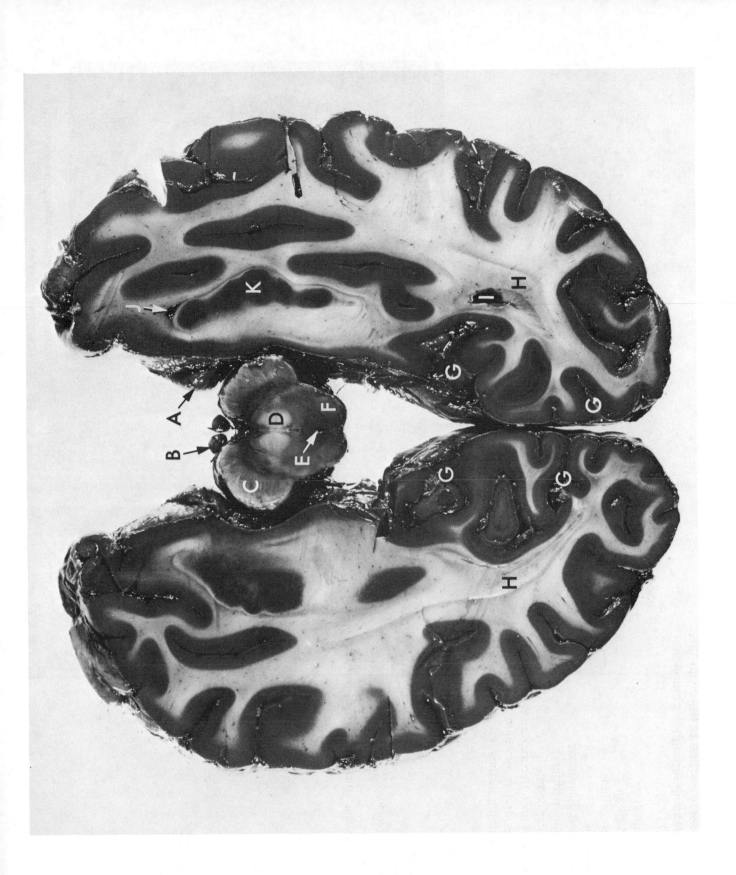

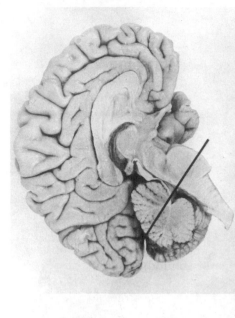

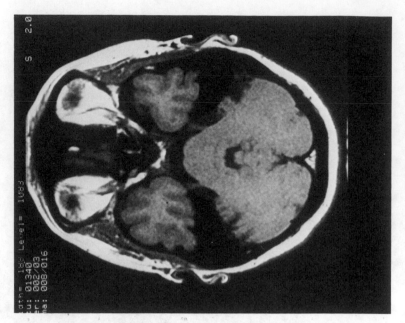

Normal T1-weighted MRI scan showing the trigeminal nerves

Figure 94 **Transverse section of the metencephalon passing through the mid-pons (or slightly below) (×3)**

A. Cerebellar hemisphere
B. Vermis of cerebellum
C. Flocculus of cerebellum
D. Fourth ventricle
E. Superior cerebellar peduncle
F. Inferior cerebellar peduncle
G. Middle cerebellar peduncle
H. Tegmentum, or posterior, part of pons
I. Basilar, or anterior, part of pons
J. Basilar artery (lying in the *basilar sulcus* of the pons)

Can you locate:

Trapezoid body
Medial lemniscus
Lateral lemniscus
Superior olivary nucleus
Pontine nuclei
Pyramidal tract (corticospinal and corticonuclear fibers)

176   *Atlas of the Brain and Spinal Cord*

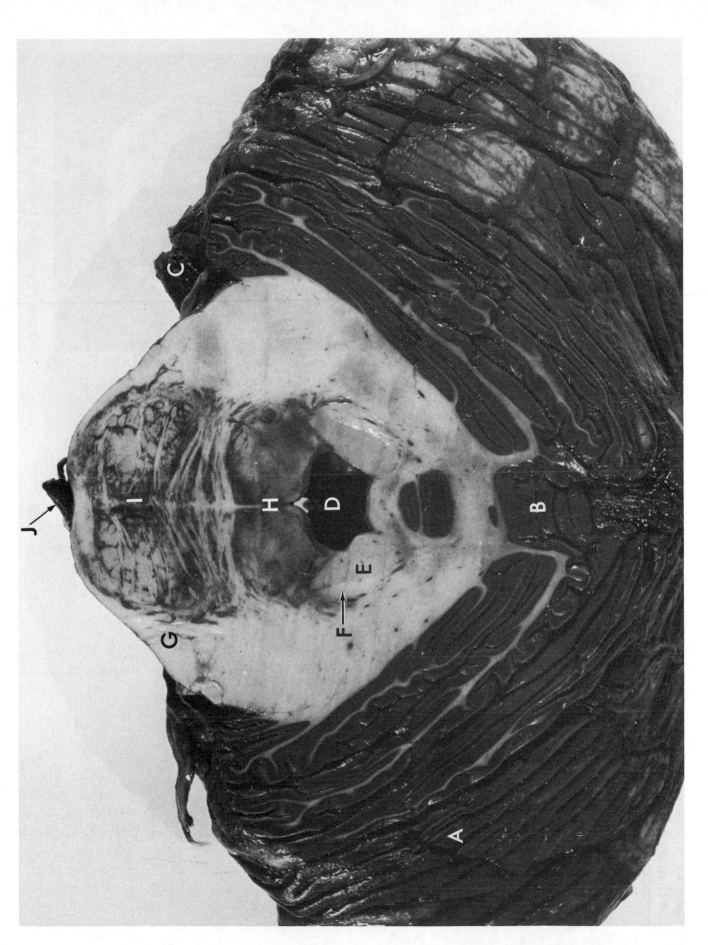

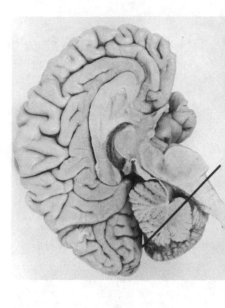

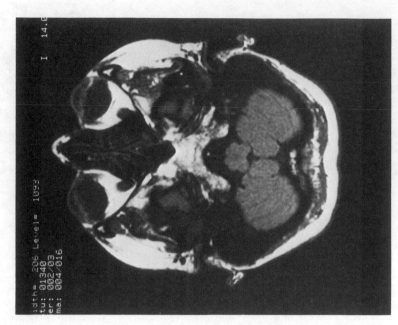

Normal T1-weighted MRI scan showing the olives and pyramids of the medulla

Figure 95 **Transverse section of the medulla and cerebellum passing through the upper portion of the medulla oblongata (×2)**

A. Cerebellar cortex (gray matter)
B. Medullary body (central white matter)
C. Cerebellar arbor vitae
D. Cerebellar folia (correspond to gyri of cerebrum)
E. Cerebellar fissures (correspond to sulci of cerebrum)
F. Dentate nucleus
G. Vermis
H. Fourth ventricle
I. Inferior olivary nucleus
J. Pyramidal tract (consists of corticospinal and corticonuclear fibers)

Can you locate:

Hypoglossal nucleus
Medial longitudinal fasciculus
Medial lemniscus
Inferior cerebellar peduncle
Inferior vestibular nucleus (and spinovestibular and vestibulospinal tracts)
Solitary tract and its nucleus
Spinal tract of trigeminal nerve (V)
Spinal nucleus of trigeminal nerve (V)

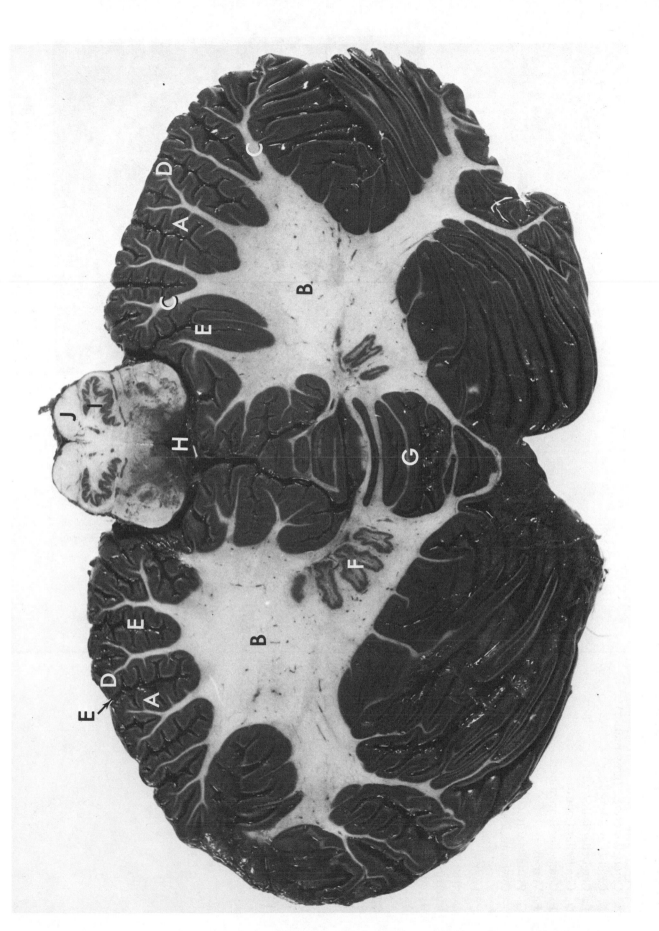

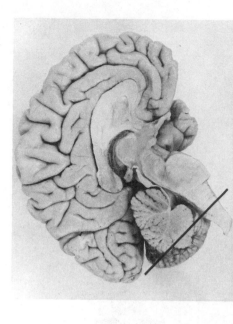

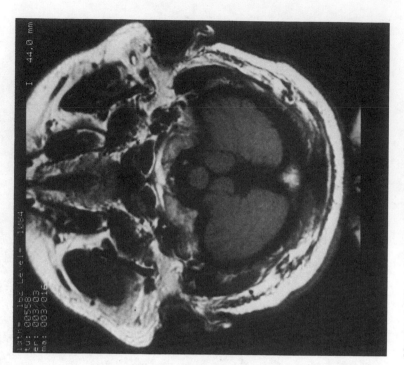

Normal T1-weighted MRI scan showing the cerebellomedullary cistern

Figure 96 **Transverse section of the medulla and cerebellum passing through the middle portion of the medulla oblongata (×2)**

A. Cerebellar cortex (gray matter)
B. Cerebellar arbor vitae
C. Cerebellar folia
D. Cerebellar fissures
E. Cerebellar hemisphere
F. Vermis
G. Pyramidal tract (consists of corticospinal and corticonuclear fibers)

Can you locate:

Nucleus and fasciculus gracilis
Nucleus and fasciculus cuneatus
Hypoglossal nucleus
Medial longitudinal fasciculus
Medial lemniscus
Spinal tract of trigeminal nerve (V)
Spinal nucleus of V

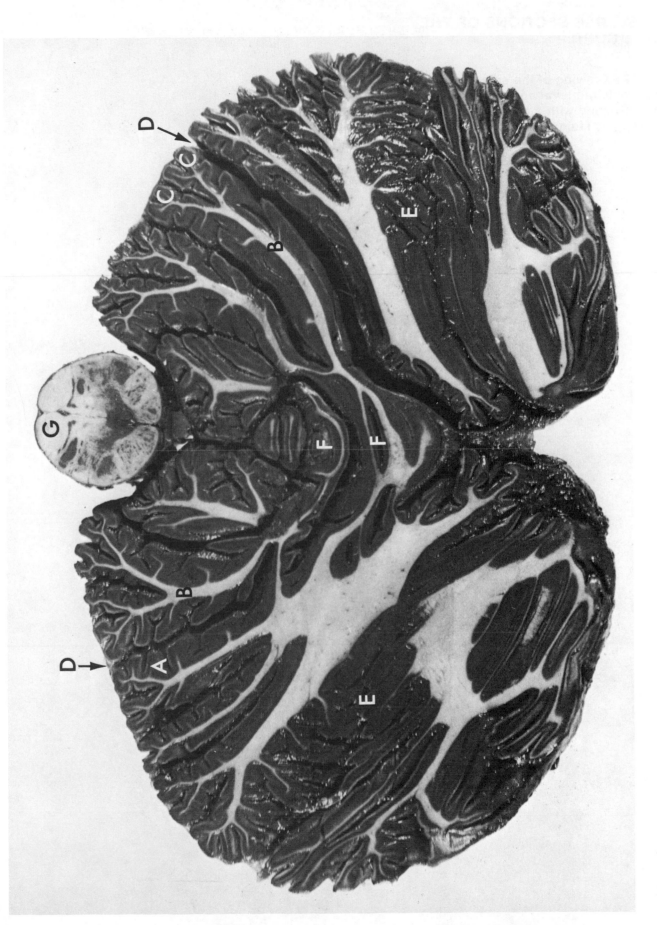

TRANSVERSE SECTIONS OF THE SPINAL CORD

Figure 97 Drawing of the spinal cord indicating the approximate level and plane of Figures 98–103 (Stained with a modification of the Weil–Weigert stain)

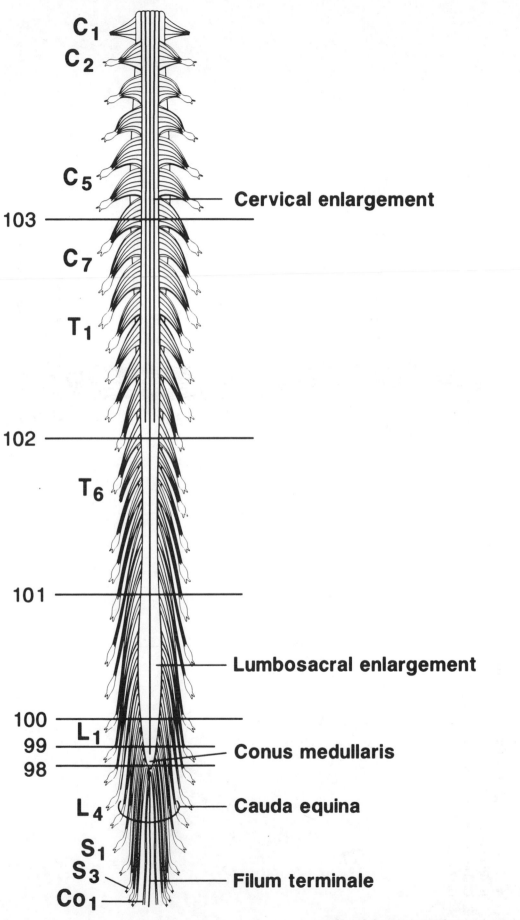

C₁

C₂

C₅

103 ——— Cervical enlargement

C₇

T₁

102 ———

T₆

101 ———

Lumbosacral enlargement

100 ———
L₁
99 ——— Conus medullaris
98 ———

L₄ Cauda equina

S₁
S₃ Filum terminale
Co₁ ———

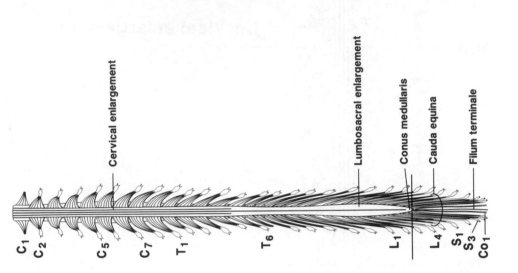

Cervical enlargement

Lumbosacral enlargement

Conus medullaris

Cauda equina

Filum terminale

C₁
C₂
C₅
C₇
T₁
T₆
L₁
L₄
S₁
S₃
Co₁

Figure 98 **Transverse section of the lowest part (conus medullaris) of the spinal cord passing through the coccygeal region of the cord and the nerve rootlets of the cauda equina (×25)**

A. Coccygeal region of the spinal cord
B. Pia mater
C. Nerve rootlets of the cauda equina
D. Arachnoid

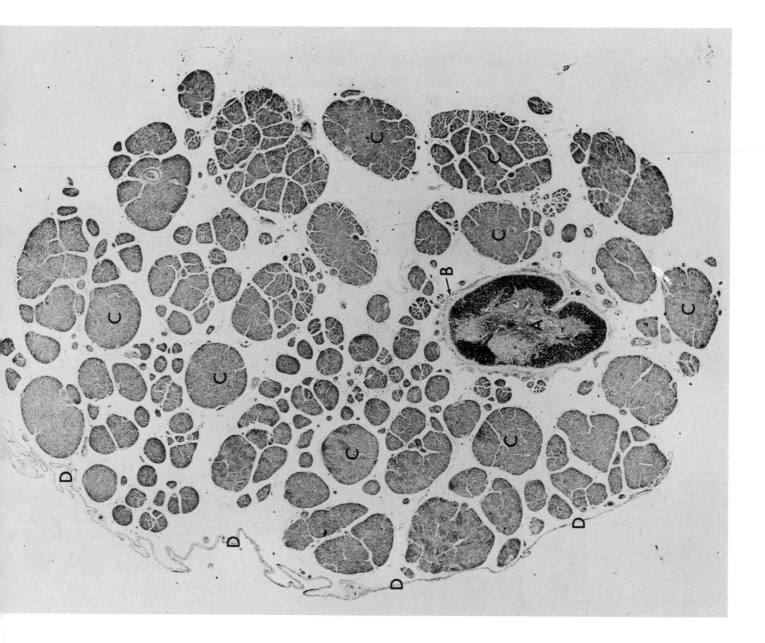

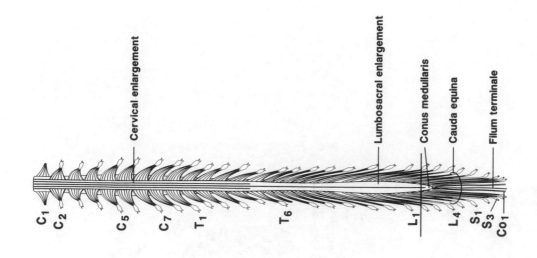

Cervical enlargement

Lumbosacral enlargement
Conus medullaris
Cauda equina
Filum terminale

C_1 C_2 C_5 C_7 T_1 T_6 L_1 L_4 S_1 S_3 Co_1

Figure 99 **Transverse section through the lower sacral region of the spinal cord (×20)**

A. Anterior spinal artery
B. Anterior spinal vein
C. Posterior spinal artery
D. Posterior spinal vein
E. Posterior funiculus (fasciculus gracilis)
F. Lateral funiculus
G. Anterior funiculus
H. Anterior horn
I. Sacral parasympathetic nucleus (in intermediate column)
J. Posterior horn

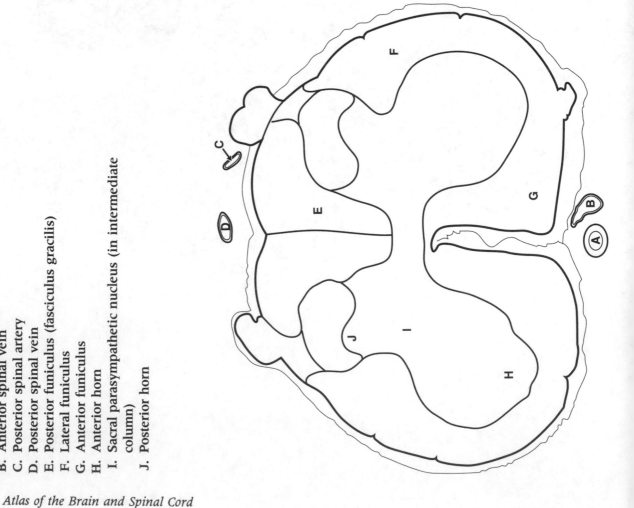

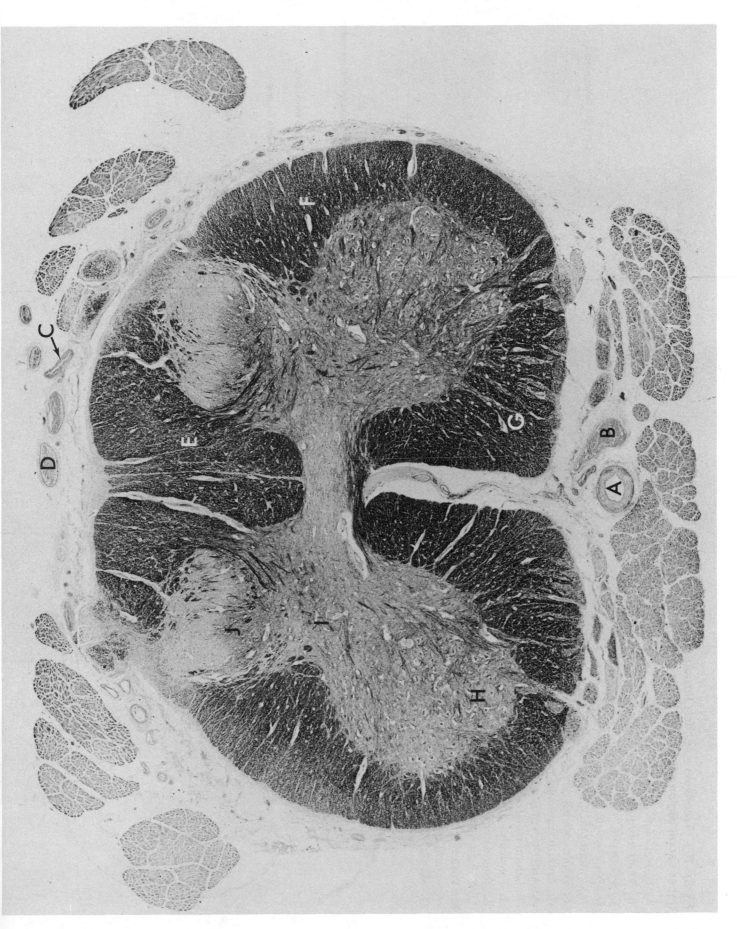

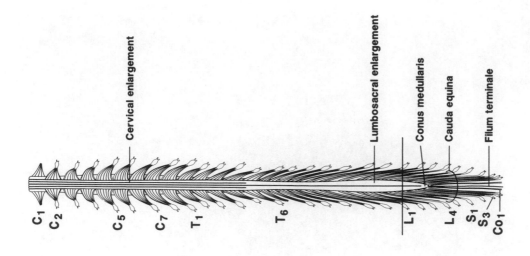

Cervical enlargement

Lumbosacral enlargement

Conus medullaris

Cauda equina

Filum terminale

C_1
C_2
C_5
C_7
T_1
T_6
L_1
L_4
S_1
S_3
Co_1

Figure 100 **Transverse section through the upper sacral region of the spinal cord (×20)**

A. Dorsal root
B. Ventral root
C. Pia mater
D. Posterior median sulcus
E. Anterior median fissure
F. White commissure
G. Anterior funiculus
H. Anterior spinocerebellar tract
I. Lateral corticospinal tract
J. Fasciculus gracilis
K. Dorsolateral tract
L. Substantia gelatinosa
M. Posterior horn nuclei
N. Lateral division of anterior horn nuclei
O. Medial division of anterior horn nuclei

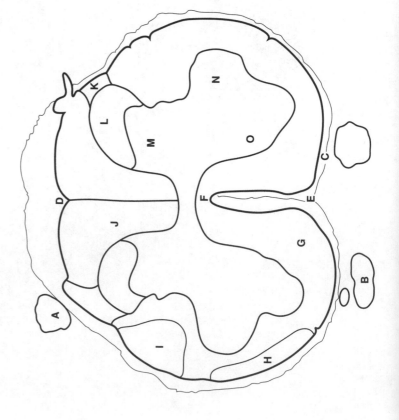

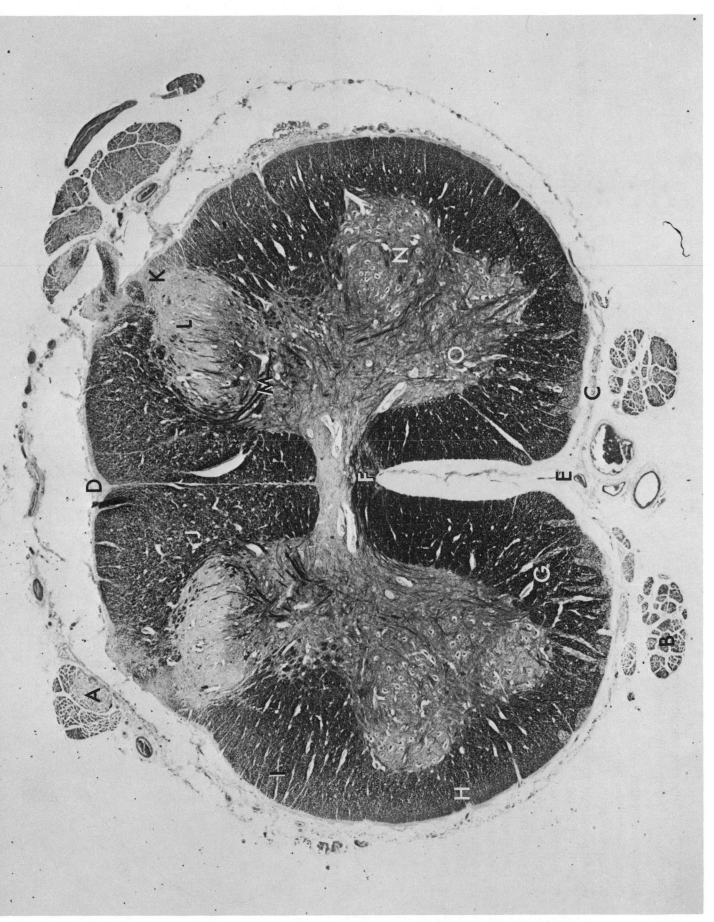

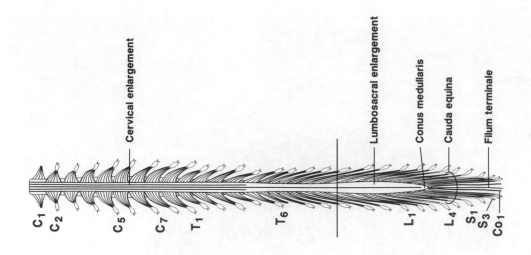

Cervical enlargement

Lumbosacral enlargement

Conus medullaris

Cauda equina

Filum terminale

C₁
C₂
C₅
C₇
T₁
T₆
L₁
L₄
S₁
S₃
Co₁

Figure 101 **Transverse section through the upper lumbar region of the spinal cord (×20)**

A. Posterior median sulcus
B. Posterior lateral sulcus
C. Anterior median fissure
D. Anterior spinal artery
E. Anterior spinal vein
F. Anterior funiculus
G. Anterior spinocerebellar tract
H. Spinothalamic tract
I. Lateral corticospinal tract
J. Fasciculus gracilis
K. Posterior horn
L. Thoracic nucleus
M. Intermediolateral and intermediomedial nuclei
N. Anterior horn

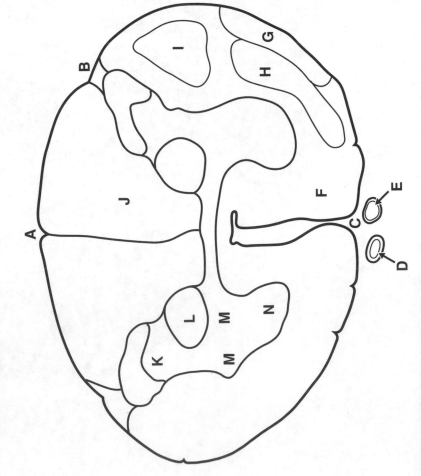

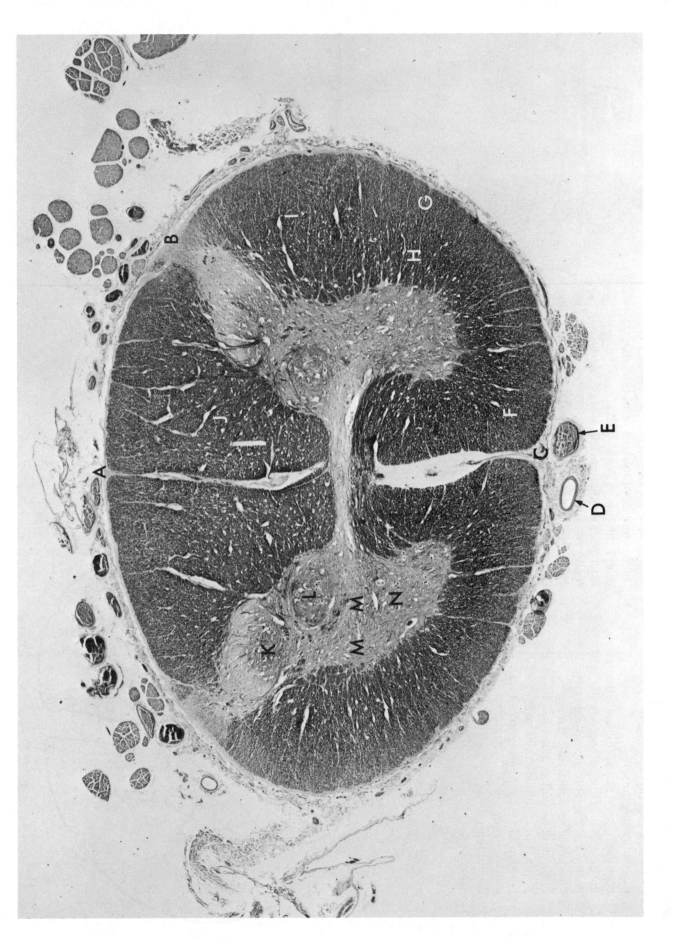

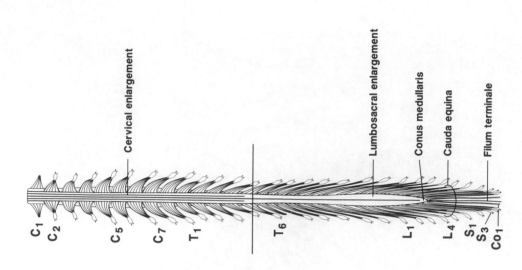

Cervical enlargement

Lumbosacral enlargement
Conus medullaris
Cauda equina
Filum terminale

C₁
C₂
C₅
C₇
T₁
T₆
L₁
L₄
S₁
S₃
Co₁

Figure 102 **Transverse section through the thoracic region of the spinal cord (×20)**

A. Fasciculus gracilis
B. Fasciculus cuneatus
C. Position of posterior spinocerebellar tract
D. Position of anterior spinocerebellar tract
E. Position of lateral corticospinal tract
F. Position of spinothalamic tract
G. Position of medullary reticulospinal tract
H. Position of vestibulospinal tract
I. Position of anterior corticospinal tract
J. Posterior horn
K. Lateral horn
L. Anterior horn

M. Medial division of anterior horn nuclei
N. Intermediolateral nucleus of intermediate (gray) column
O. Intermediomedial nucleus of intermediate (gray) column
P. Thoracic nucleus (nucl. dorsalis, Clarke's nucl.)
Q. Central canal
R. Position of pontine reticulospinal tract

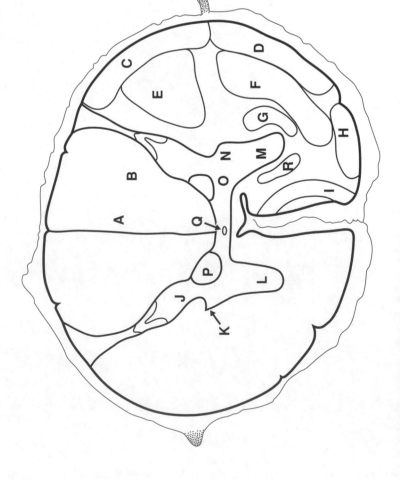

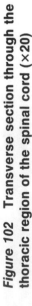

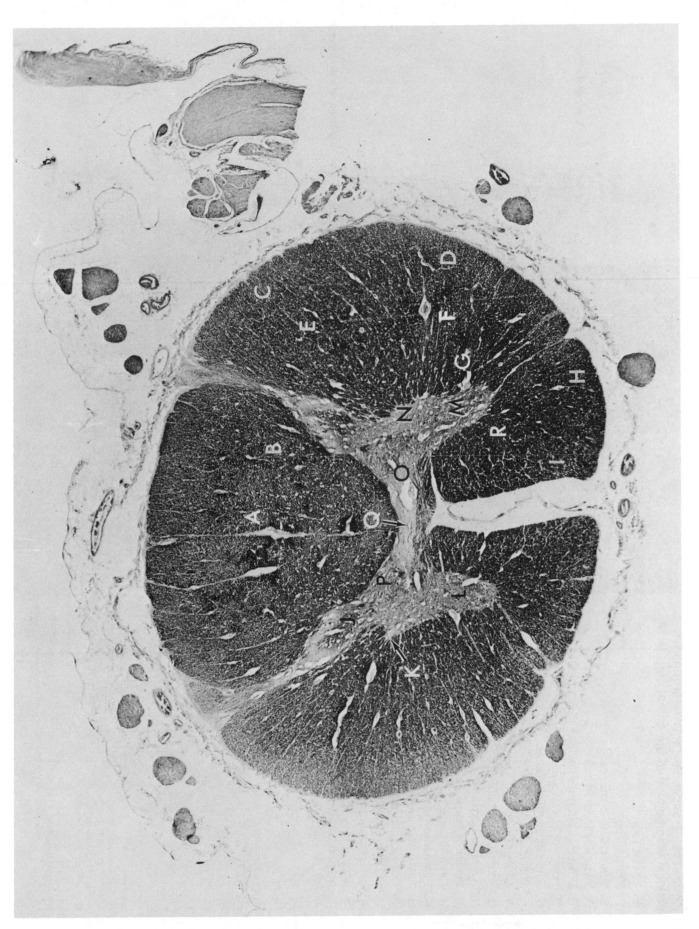

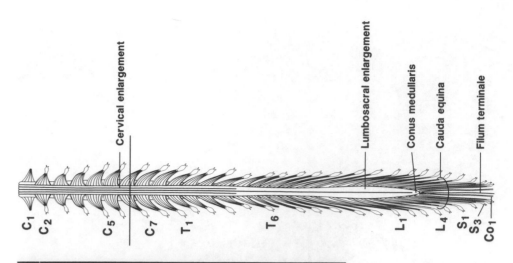

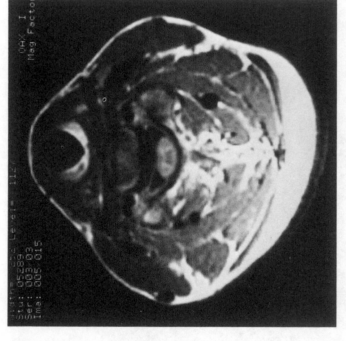

Normal T1-weighted MRI scan of the cervical spinal cord

Figure 103 **Transverse section through the cervical enlargement of the spinal cord (×18)**

A. Dorsal root
B. Ventral root
C. Denticulate ligament
D. Posterior median sulcus
E. Posterior intermediate sulcus
F. Posterior lateral sulcus
G. Anterior median fissure
H. Posterior funiculus
I. Lateral funiculus
J. Anterior funiculus
K. Anterior horn
L. Posterior horn
M. Central canal
N. Fasciculus gracilis
O. Fasciculus cuneatus
P. Dorsolateral tract (Lissauer)
Q. Substantia gelatinosa
R. Posterior horn nuclei
S. Lateral division of anterior horn nuclei
T. Medial division of anterior horn nuclei

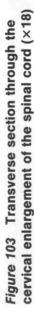

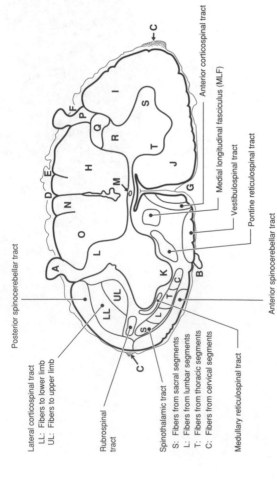

Posterior spinocerebellar tract

Lateral corticospinal tract
LL: Fibers to lower limb
UL: Fibers to upper limb

Rubrospinal tract

Spinothalamic tract
S: Fibers from sacral segments
L: Fibers from lumbar segments
T: Fibers from thoracic segments
C: Fibers from cervical segments

Medullary reticulospinal tract

Anterior spinocerebellar tract

Pontine reticulospinal tract

Vestibulospinal tract

Medial longitudinal fasciculus (MLF)

Anterior corticospinal tract

Cervical enlargement

Lumbosacral enlargement
Conus medullaris
Cauda equina
Filum terminale

C1
C2
C5
C7
T1
T6
L1
L4
S1
S3
Co1

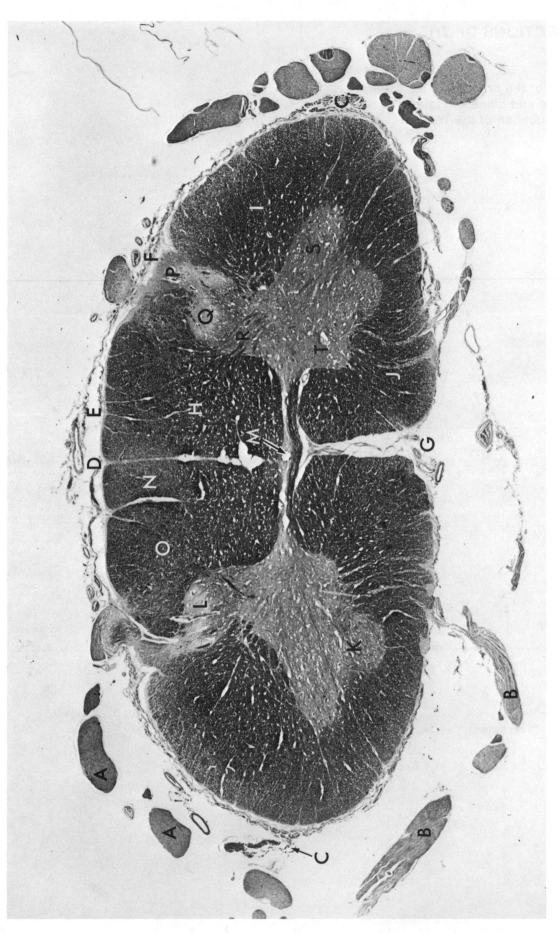

TRANSVERSE SECTIONS OF THE BRAIN STEM

Figure 104   Drawing of the brain stem indicating the approximate level and plane of Figures 105–117 (Loyez modification of the Weigert stain)

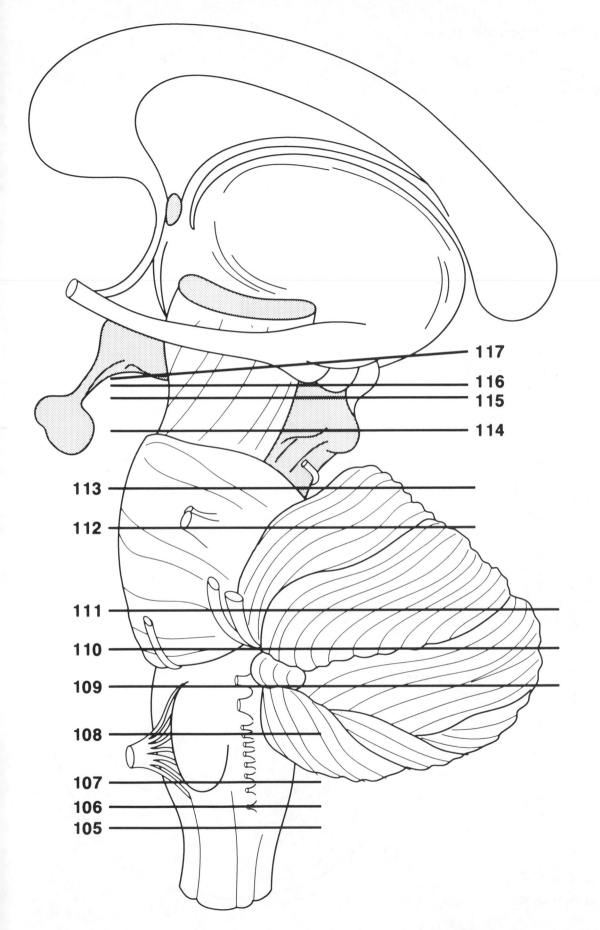

117

116
115

114

113

112

111

110

109

108

107
106
105

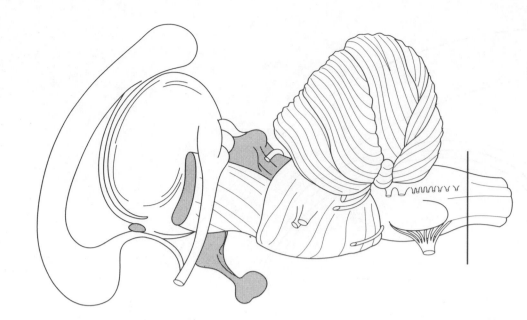

Figure 105 Transverse section of the transition from medulla to spinal cord passing through the decussation of the pyramidal tracts (×18)

A. Pia mater
B. Nucleus gracilis
C. Fasciculus gracilis
D. Fasciculus cuneatus
E. Spinal tract of trigeminal nerve (V)
F. Spinal nucleus of V
G. Posterior spinocerebellar tract
H. Anterior spinocerebellar tract

I. Anterior horn of spinal cord
J. Medial longitudinal fasciculus
K. Anterior corticospinal tract
L. Pyramidal decussation
M. Lateral corticospinal tract
N. Central canal
O. Spinal lemniscus (contains spinothalamic tract and spinotectal tract)

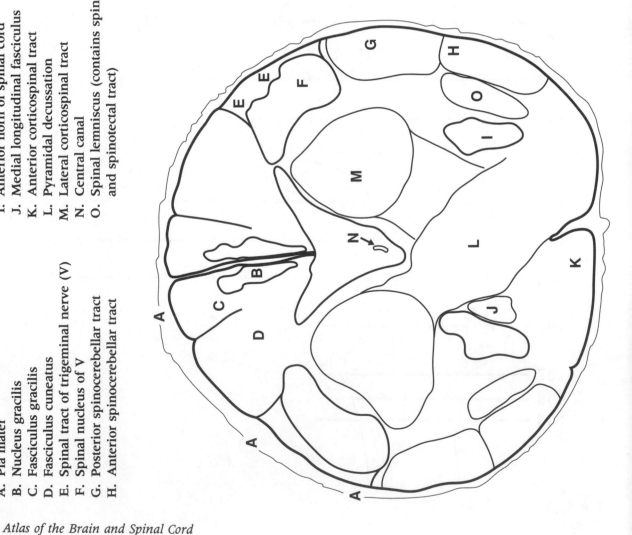

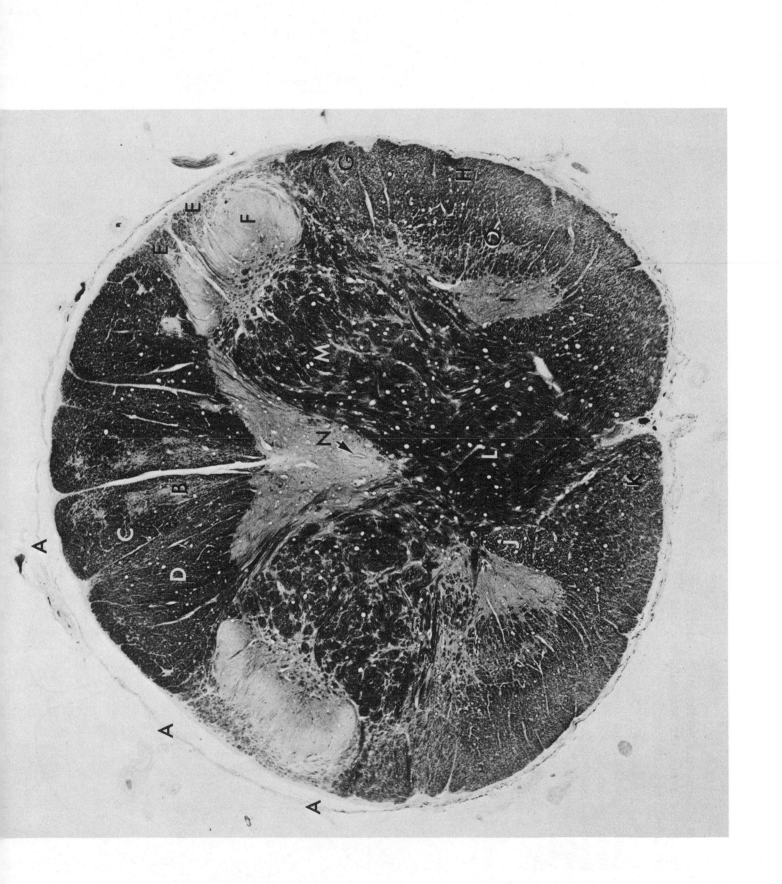

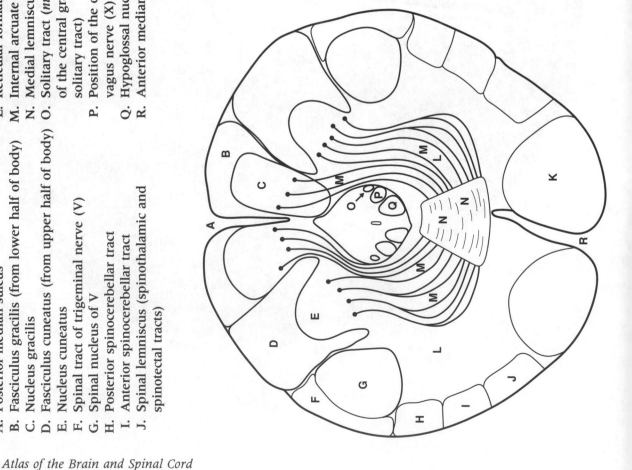

Figure 106 **Transverse section of the lower medulla at the level of the decussation of the medial lemniscus (×16)**

A. Posterior median sulcus
B. Fasciculus gracilis (from lower half of body)
C. Nucleus gracilis
D. Fasciculus cuneatus (from upper half of body)
E. Nucleus cuneatus
F. Spinal tract of trigeminal nerve (V)
G. Spinal nucleus of V
H. Posterior spinocerebellar tract
I. Anterior spinocerebellar tract
J. Spinal lemniscus (spinothalamic and spinotectal tracts)
K. Pyramidal tract
L. Reticular formation
M. Internal arcuate fibers
N. Medial lemniscus and its decussation
O. Solitary tract (*nucleus of solitary tract is that part of the central gray substance surrounding the solitary tract*)
P. Position of the dorsal (motor) nucleus of the vagus nerve (X)
Q. Hypoglossal nucleus
R. Anterior median fissure

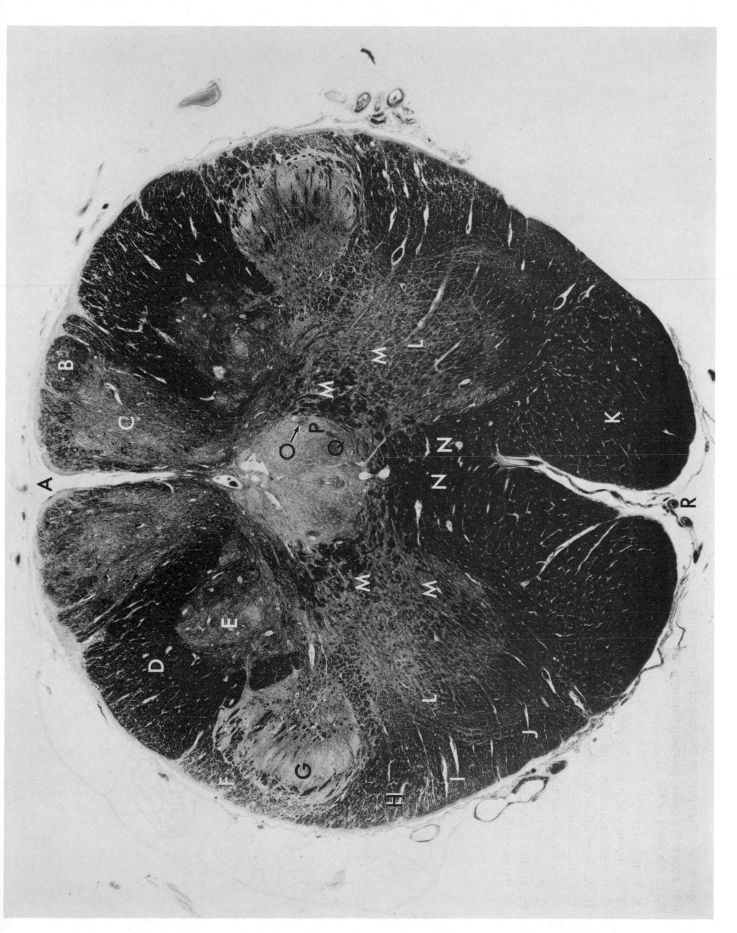

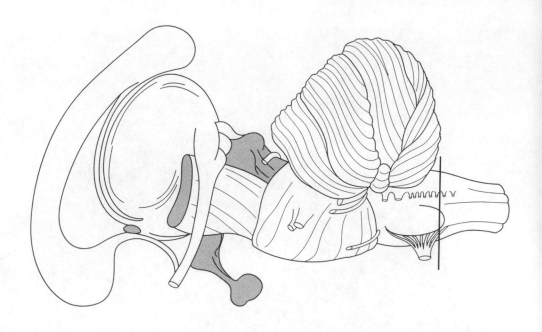

Figure 107 **Transverse section of the medulla, just above the obex, passing through the lower tip of the olive (×12)**

A. Fourth ventricle
B. Fasciculus and nucleus cuneatus
C. Posterior spinocerebellar tract
D. Anterior spinocerebellar tract
E. Spinal lemniscus
F. Inferior olivary nucleus
G. Pyramidal tract
H. Medial lemniscus
I. Hypoglossal nucleus

J. Dorsal longitudinal fasciculus
K. Dorsal (motor) nucleus of the vagus nerve (X)
L. Solitary tract (*nucleus of solitary tract is the gray matter surrounding the tract*)
M. Reticular formation
N. Medial longitudinal fasciculus (MLF)
O. Spinal tract of trigeminal nerve (V)
P. Spinal nucleus of V

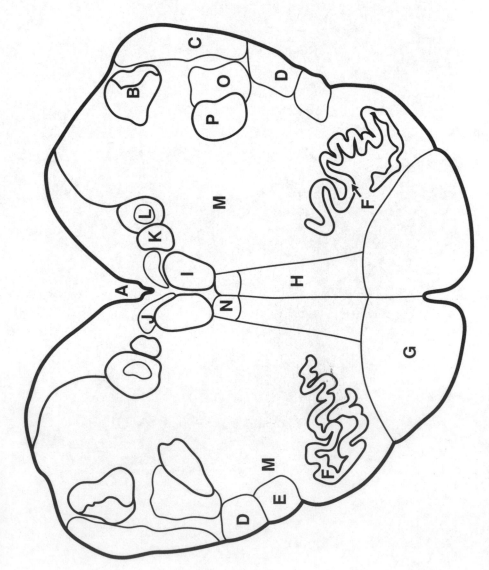

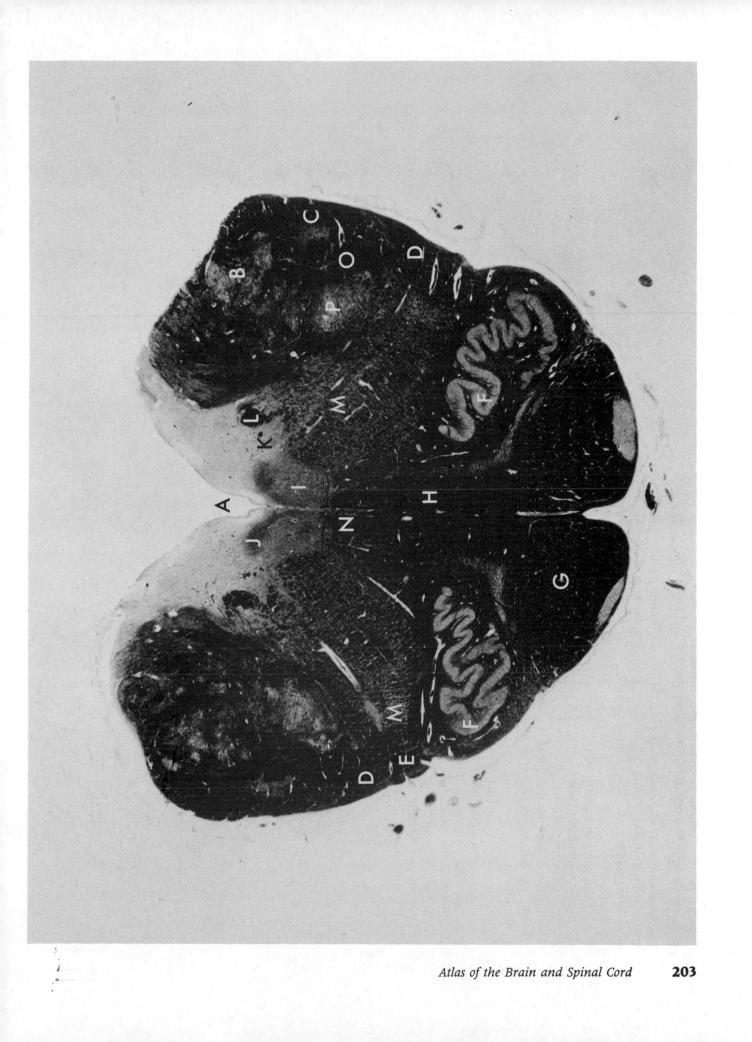

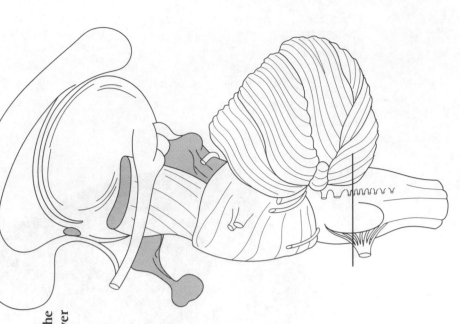

Figure 108 Transverse section of the medulla passing through the middle of the olive (×12)

A. Choroid plexus of fourth ventricle
B. Inferior medullary velum
C. Fourth ventricle
D. Pia mater
E. Inferior cerebellar peduncle
F. Spinal tract of trigeminal nerve (V)
G. Spinal nucleus of V
H. Position of nucleus ambiguus
I. Anterior spinocerebellar tract and spinal lemniscus
J. Inferior olivary nucleus (forms the external bulge known as the *olive*)
K. Pyramidal tract (forms the external bulge known as the *pyramid*)
L. Medial lemniscus
M. Hypoglossal nucleus
N. Dorsal (motor) nucleus of the vagus nerve (X)

O. Solitary tract
P. Nucleus of the solitary tract
Q. Medial vestibular nucleus
R. Inferior vestibular nucleus (and spinovestibular and vestibulospinal tracts)
S. Accessory cuneate nucleus
T. Reticular formation (*nucleus gigantocellularis*)
U. Medial longitudinal fasciculus (MLF)
V. Cuneate part of medial lemniscus (from upper half of body)
W. Gracile part of medial lemniscus (from lower half of body)
X. Fibers of hypoglossal nerve (XII)
Y. Fibers of vagus nerve (X)
Z. Position of fibers in the pyramidal tract to the face (F), upper limb (U), trunk (T), and lower limb (L), as indicated in the drawing

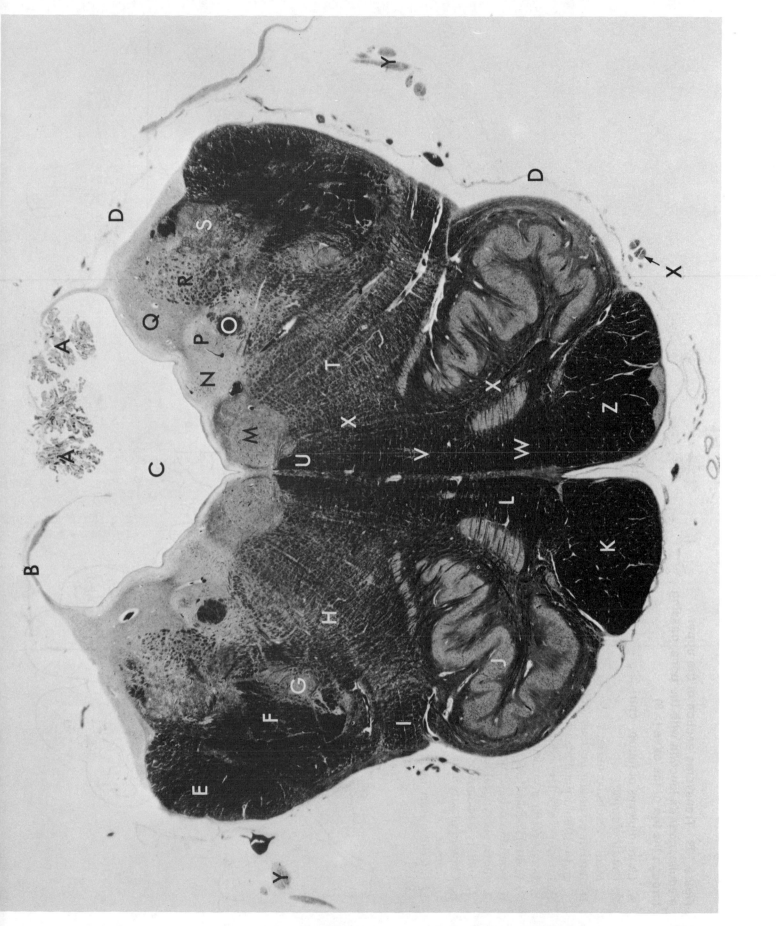

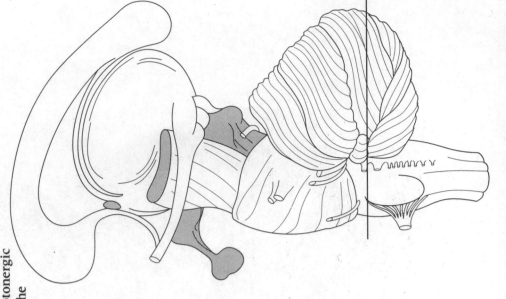

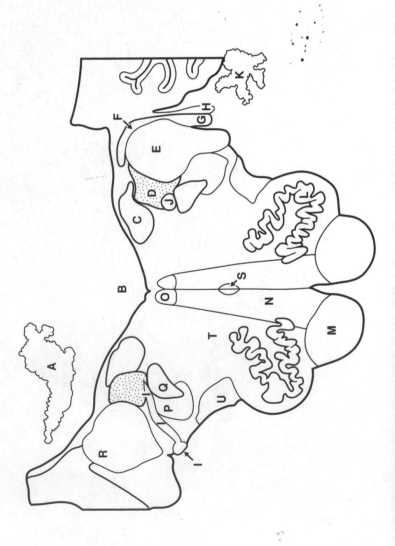

Figure 109 **Transverse section of the upper medulla, near its junction with the pons, passing through the top of the olive (×8)**

A. Choroid plexus of fourth ventricle
B. Fourth ventricle
C. Medial vestibular nucleus
D. Inferior vestibular nucleus (and spinovestibular and vestibulospinal tracts)
E. Inferior cerebellar peduncle
F. Dorsal cochlear nucleus
G. Ventral cochlear nucleus
H. Vestibulocochlear nerve (VIII), cochlear part
I. Glossopharyngeal nerve (IX)
J. Solitary tract and its nucleus
K. Choroid plexus in the *lateral recess of the fourth ventricle*
L. Inferior olivary nucleus

M. Pyramidal tract
N. Medial lemniscus
O. Medial longitudinal fasciculus (MLF)
P. Spinal tract of trigeminal nerve (V)
Q. Spinal nucleus of V
R. Inferior cerebellar peduncle entering the cerebellum
S. Reticular formation (*nucleus raphe magnus,* which is a source of descending serotonergic projections to the posterior horn of the spinal cord for pain modulation)
T. Reticular formation (*nucleus gigantocellularis*)
U. Spinal lemniscus

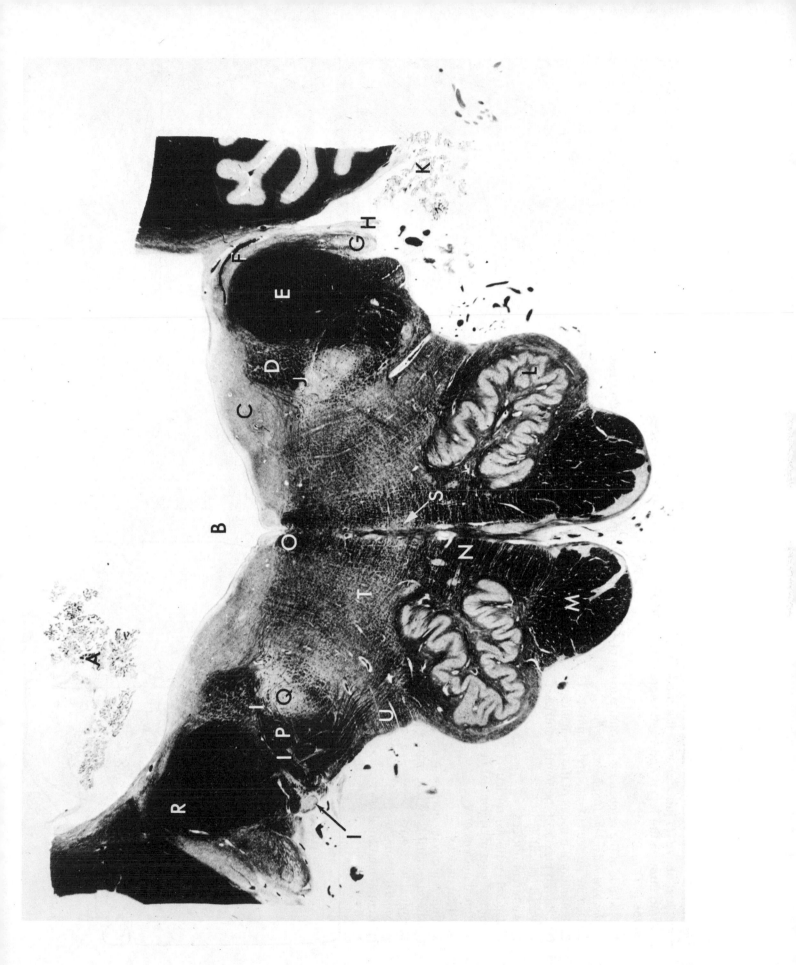

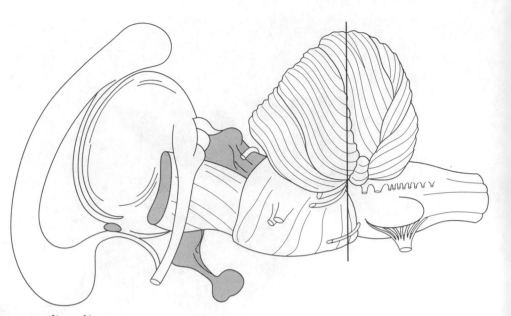

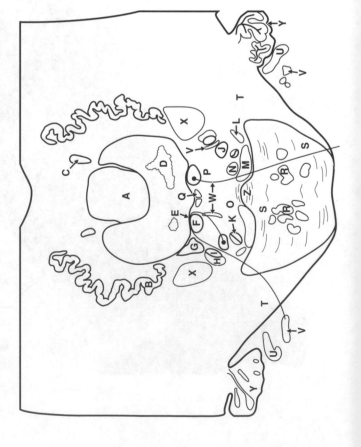

Figure 110 Transverse section of the lower pons, just above its junction with the medulla, passing through the facial and vestibulocochlear nerves (×7)

A. Nodulus of the cerebellum [vermal portion of *flocculonodular lobe (vestibulocerebellum)*]
B. Dentate nucleus of the cerebellum
C. Emboliform nucleus of the cerebellum
D. Choroid plexus of the fourth ventricle
E. Facial colliculus
F. Abducent nucleus
G. Lateral vestibular nucleus
H. Spinal tract of trigeminal nerve (V)
I. Spinal nucleus of V
J. Facial nucleus
K. Superior olivary nucleus (gray matter) and lateral lemniscus (white matter)
L. Spinal lemniscus
M. Medial lemniscus
N. Central tegmental tract

O. Reticular formation (*nucleus reticularis pontis caudalis*)
P. Paramedian pontine reticular formation (PPRF)
Q. Medial longitudinal fasciculus (MLF)
R. Pyramidal tract
S. Pontine nuclei
T. Middle cerebellar peduncle
U. Vestibulocochlear nerve (VIII)
V. Facial nerve (VII)
W. Fibers of the abducent nerve (VI)
X. Inferior cerebellar peduncle (entering the cerebellum)
Y. Flocculus of the cerebellum [hemispheric portion of *flocculonodular lobe (vestibulocerebellum)*]
Z. Trapezoid body (crossing fibers)

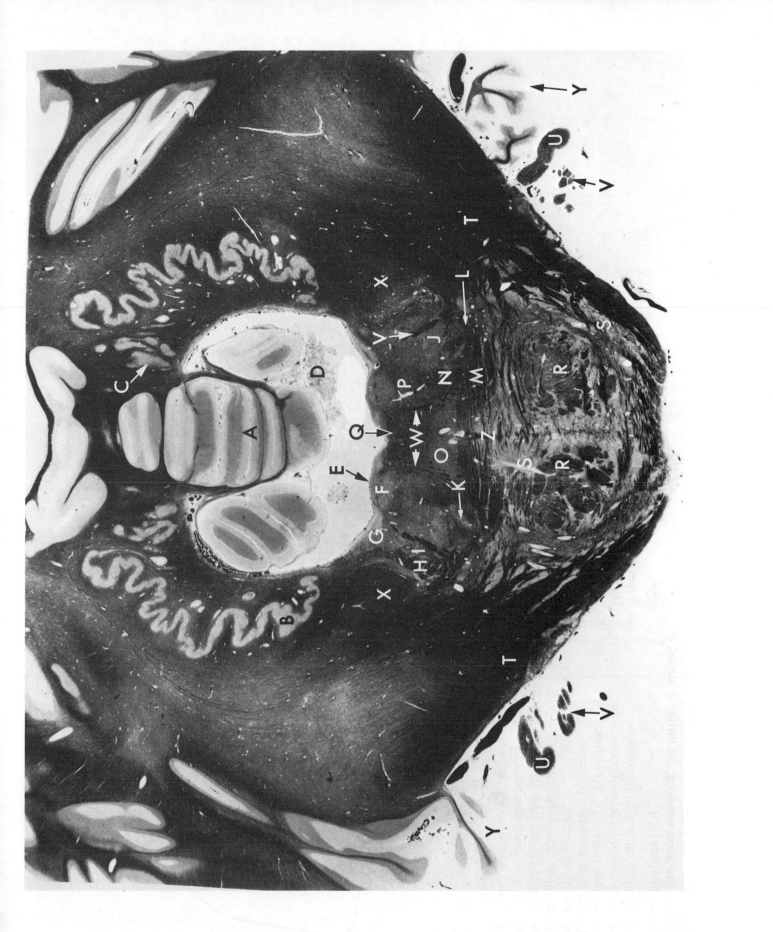

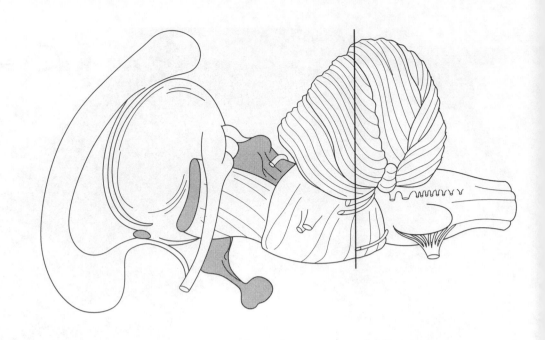

Figure 111 Transverse section of the lower third of the pons showing the intrinsic nuclei of the cerebellum (×6)

A. Fastigial nucleus of cerebellum
B. Emboliform nucleus of cerebellum
C. Dentate nucleus of cerebellum
D. Superior cerebellar peduncle
E. Fourth ventricle
F. Genu of facial nerve (VII)
G. Medial longitudinal fasciculus (MLF)
H. Superior vestibular nucleus
I. Spinal tract of trigeminal nerve (V) and its
   nucleus

J. Superior olivary nucleus (gray matter) and
   lateral lemniscus (white matter)
K. Spinal lemniscus
L. Medial lemniscus
M. Trapezoid body
N. Central tegmental tract
O. Reticular formation
P. Pyramidal tract
Q. Pontine nuclei
R. Middle cerebellar peduncle

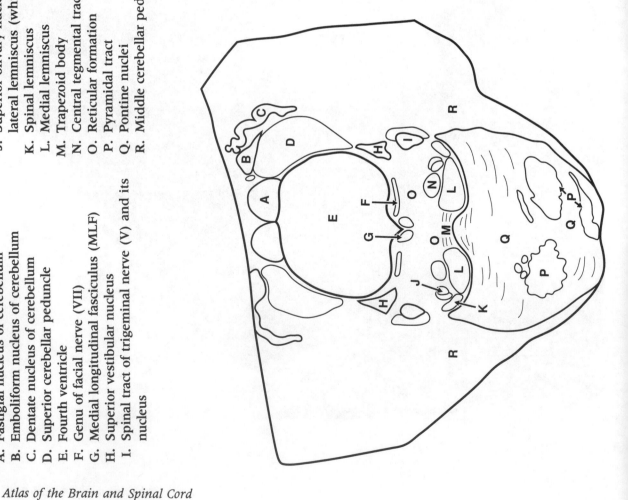

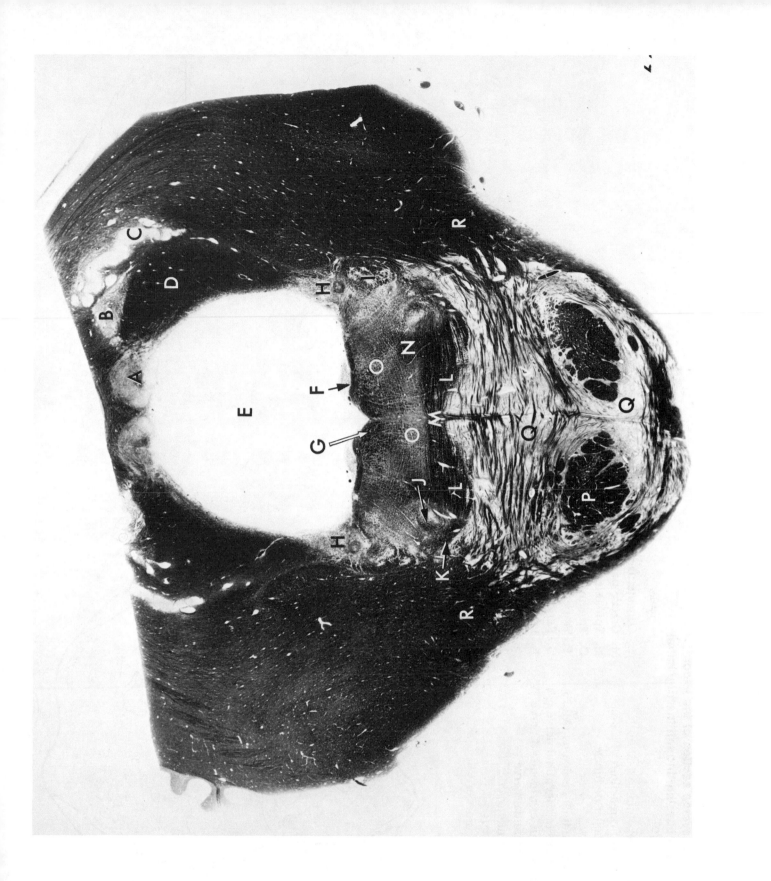

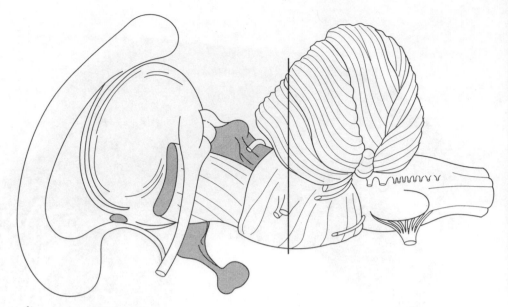

Figure 112 **Transverse section of the middle third of the pons passing through the trigeminal nerve (×6)**

A. Vermis of cerebellum
B. Hemisphere of cerebellum
C. Superior cerebellar peduncle
D. Fourth ventricle
E. Medial longitudinal fasciculus (MLF)
F. Motor nucleus of trigeminal nerve (V)
G. Pontine nucleus of trigeminal nerve (V)
H. Fibers of trigeminal nerve (V)
I. Central tegmental tract
J. Medial lemniscus
K. Mesencephalic tract of V

L. Cuneate part of medial lemniscus
M. Gracile part of medial lemniscus
N. Spinal lemniscus
O. Trigeminal lemniscus (trigeminothalamic tract)
P. Trapezoid body
Q. Reticular formation
R. Pyramidal tract and corticopontine fibers
S. Pontine nuclei
T. Middle cerebellar peduncle
U. Basilar artery (lying in the *basilar sulcus of the pons*)

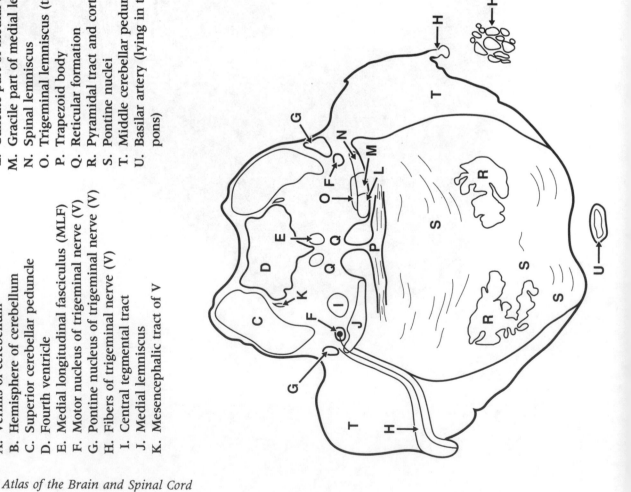

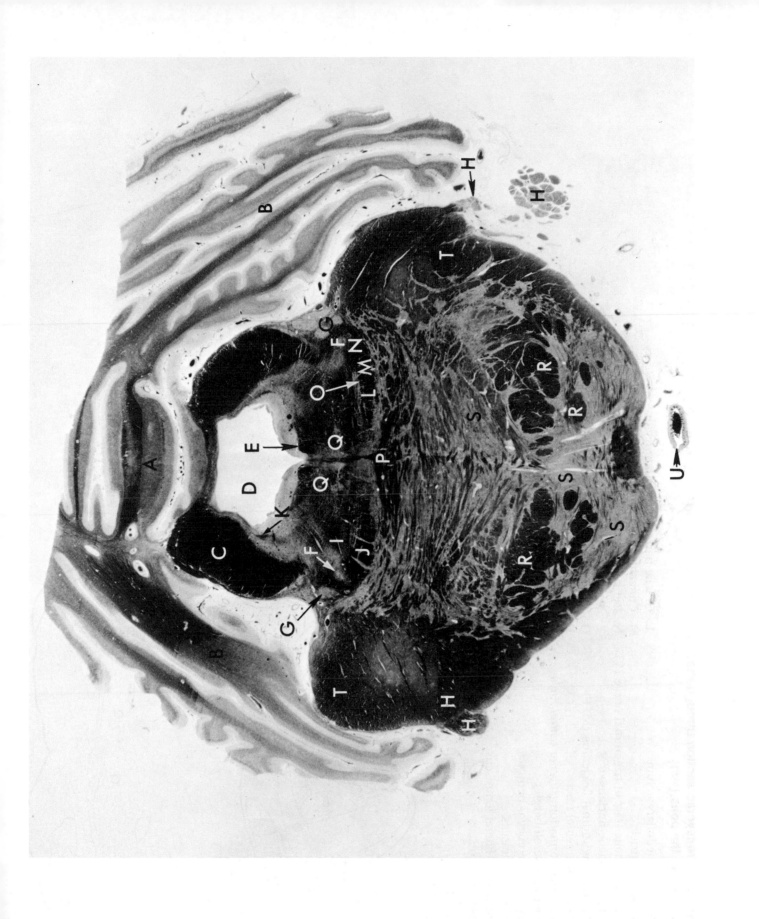

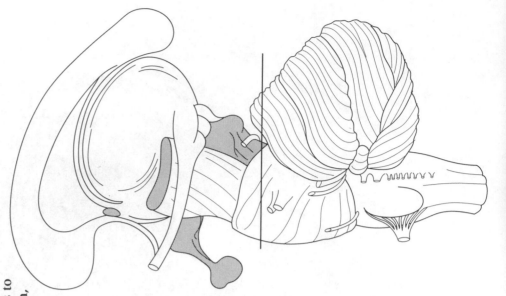

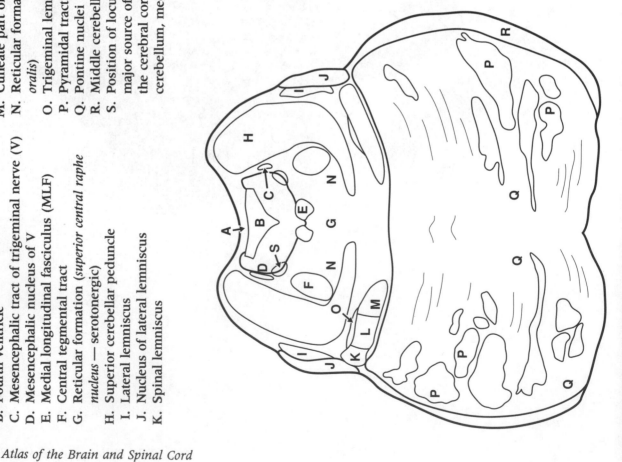

Figure 113 **Transverse section through the upper third of the pons (×8)**

A. Superior medullary velum
B. Fourth ventricle
C. Mesencephalic tract of trigeminal nerve (V)
D. Mesencephalic nucleus of V
E. Medial longitudinal fasciculus (MLF)
F. Central tegmental tract
G. Reticular formation (*superior central raphe nucleus* — serotonergic)
H. Superior cerebellar peduncle
I. Lateral lemniscus
J. Nucleus of lateral lemniscus
K. Spinal lemniscus
L. Gracile part of medial lemniscus
M. Cuneate part of medial lemniscus
N. Reticular formation (*nucleus reticularis pontis oralis*)
O. Trigeminal lemniscus
P. Pyramidal tract and corticopontine fibers
Q. Pontine nuclei
R. Middle cerebellar peduncle
S. Position of locus ceruleus (this nucleus is a major source of norepinephrine projections to the cerebral cortex, diencephalon, midbrain, cerebellum, medulla, and spinal cord)

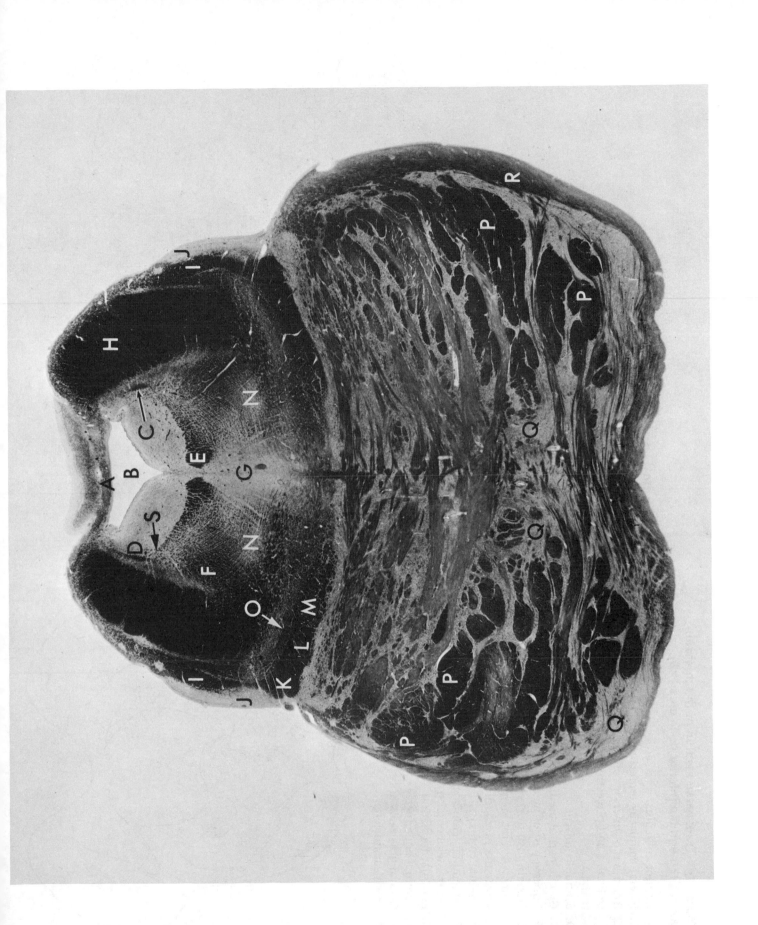

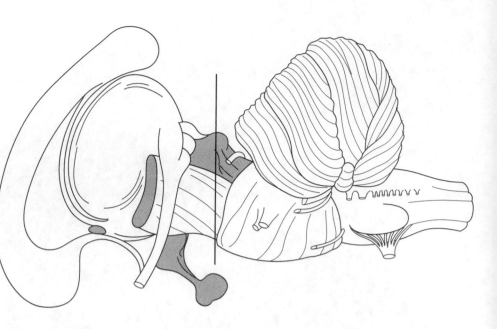

Figure 114 **Transverse section of the midbrain passing through the inferior colliculus (×8)**

A. Inferior colliculus
B. Lateral lemniscus (entering inferior colliculus)
C. Brachium of inferior colliculus (leaving inferior colliculus and projecting to medial geniculate body)
D. Spinal lemniscus
E. Gracile part of medial lemniscus
F. Cuneate part of medial lemniscus
G. Dorsal (posterior) nucleus of raphe (a major source of serotonergic projections to the substantia nigra, diencephalon, striatum, and cerebral cortex)
H. Trigeminal lemniscus
I. Central tegmental tract
J. Reticular formation
K. Cerebral aqueduct
L. Central gray substance
M. Trochlear nucleus

N. Medial longitudinal fasciculus (MLF)
O. Decussation of superior cerebellar peduncles
P. Substantia nigra (a major source of dopaminergic projections to the striatum)
Q. Crus cerebri
R. Frontopontine tract
S. Corticonuclear (corticobulbar) fibers of the pyramidal tract, eventually supplying muscles of the face, pharynx, larynx, tongue, etc.
T. Corticospinal fibers of the pyramidal tract supplying the upper limb
U. Corticospinal fibers of the pyramidal tract supplying the trunk
V. Corticospinal fibers of the pyramidal tract supplying the lower limb
W. Temporoparieto-occipitopontine tract
X. Interpeduncular fossa

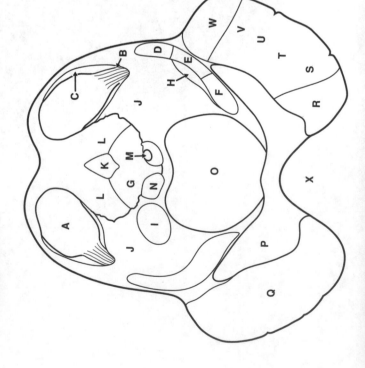

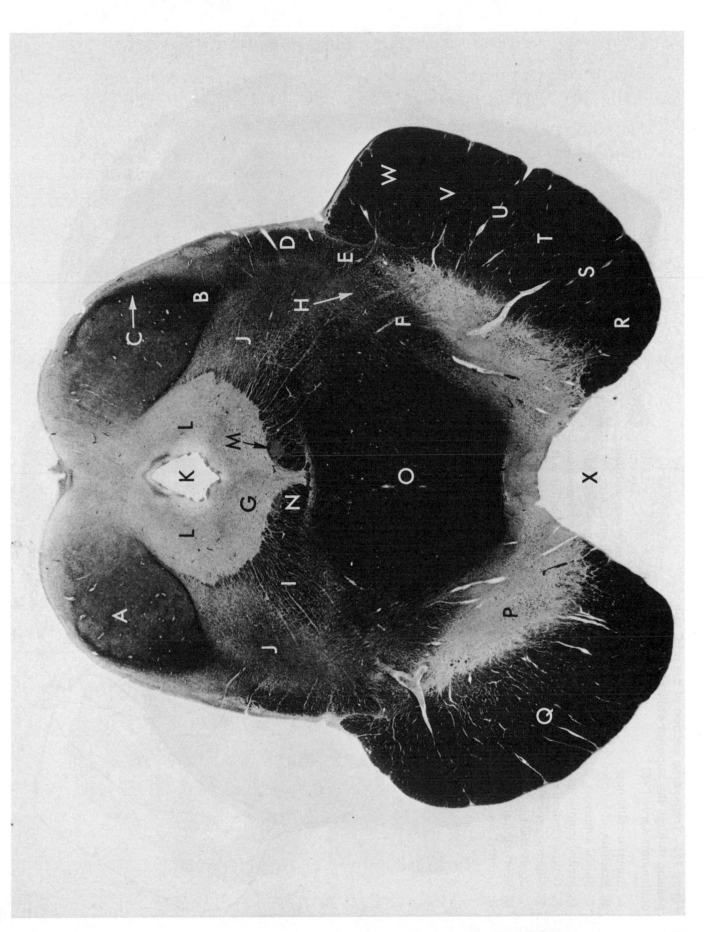

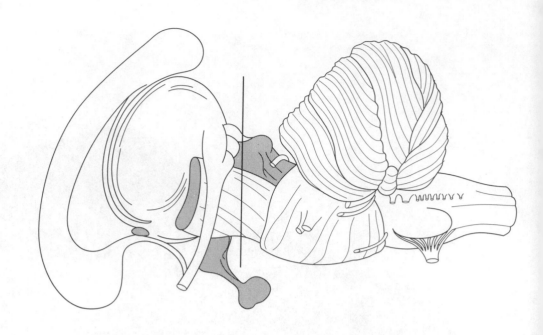

Figure 115 Transverse section of the midbrain passing through the superior colliculus and the oculomotor nerve (×8)

A. Superior colliculus
B. Brachium of inferior colliculus
C. Spinal lemniscus
D. Medial lemniscus
E. Central tegmental tract
F. Superior cerebellar peduncle (above decussation)
G. Reticular formation
H. Cerebral aqueduct
I. Central gray substance
J. Position of accessory oculomotor nucleus (Edinger–Westphal)
K. Oculomotor nucleus
L. Medial longitudinal fasciculus (MLF)
M. Fibers of oculomotor nerves (III)
N. Substantia nigra (dopaminergic)
O. Crus cerebri
P. Interpeduncular fossa

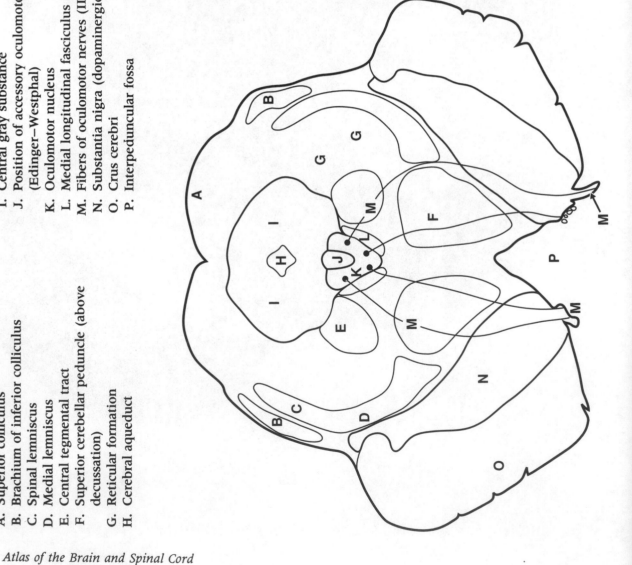

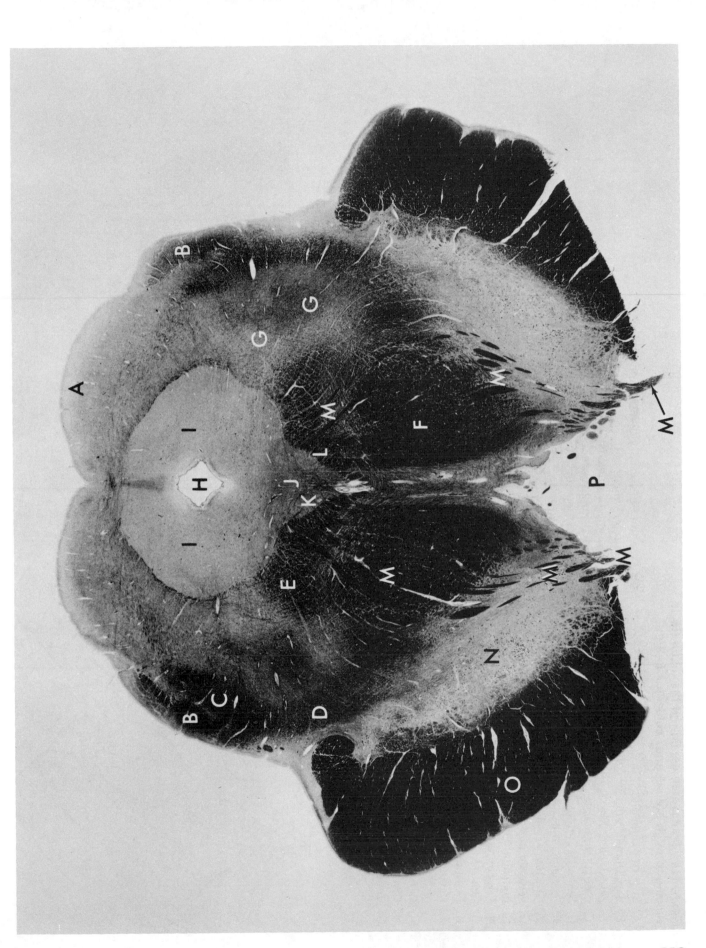

Figure 116 **Transverse section of the midbrain passing through the superior colliculus (×8)**

A. Superior colliculus
B. Brachium of inferior colliculus (entering medial geniculate body on the right)
C. Medial geniculate body of the thalamus
D. Reticular formation
E. Spinal lemniscus
F. Gracile part of medial lemniscus
G. Cuneate part of medial lemniscus
H. Substantia nigra (pars reticularis)
I. Trigeminal lemniscus
J. Central tegmental tract
K. Red nucleus
L. Habenulopeduncular tract (fasciculus retroflexus)
M. Dentatorubrothalamic tract
N. Cerebral aqueduct
O. Central gray substance

P. Position of accessory oculomotor nucleus (Edinger–Westphal)
Q. Oculomotor nucleus
R. Medial longitudinal fasciculus (MLF)
S. Fibers of oculomotor nerves (III) (difficult to see)
T. Substantia nigra (pars compacta)
U. Frontopontine tract
V. Corticonuclear (corticobulbar) fibers of pyramidal tract to face and head and neck
W. Corticospinal fibers of pyramidal tract to upper limb
X. Corticospinal fibers of pyramidal tract to trunk and lower limb
Y. Temporoparieto-occipitopontine tract
Z. Crus cerebri

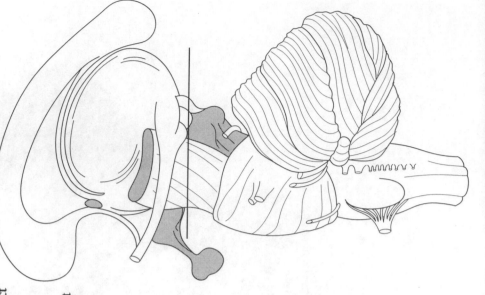

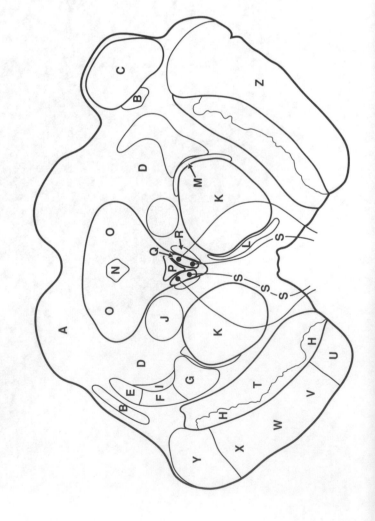

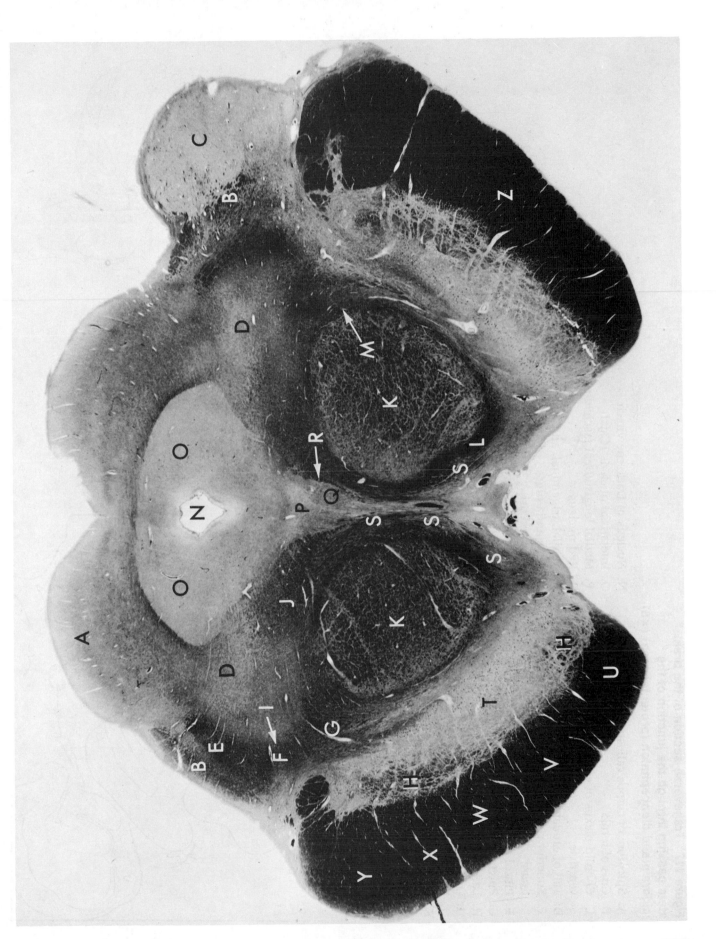

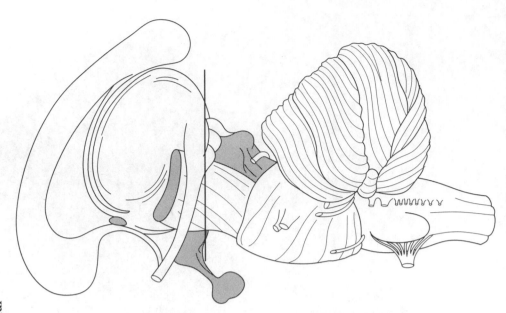

Figure 117 Transverse section of the brain stem passing through the junction of the midbrain and diencephalon (pretectal area) (×6)

A. Splenium of corpus callosum
B. Crus of fornix
C. Choroid plexus of central part of lateral ventricle
D. Tail of caudate nucleus
E. Superior cistern within the *transverse cerebral fissure*
F. Pineal body
G. Pulvinar of thalamus
H. Lateral geniculate body
I. Optic tract
J. Medial geniculate body
K. Pretectal area
L. Posterior commissure
M. Cerebral aqueduct (surrounded by the *central gray substance*)
N. Nucleus of Darkschewitsch
O. Interstitial nucleus (Cajal)
P. Medial longitudinal fasciculus (MLF)
Q. Red nucleus
R. Medial, trigeminal, and spinal lemnisci
S. Substantia nigra
T. Crus cerebri
U. Choroid plexus of inferior horn of lateral ventricle
V. Inferior horn of lateral ventricle
W. Hippocampus
X. Uncal sulcus
Y. Parahippocampal gyrus
Z. Posterior cerebral arteries

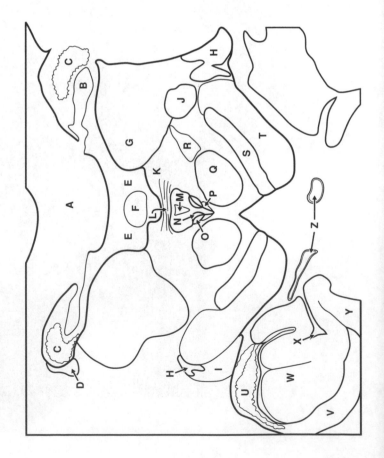

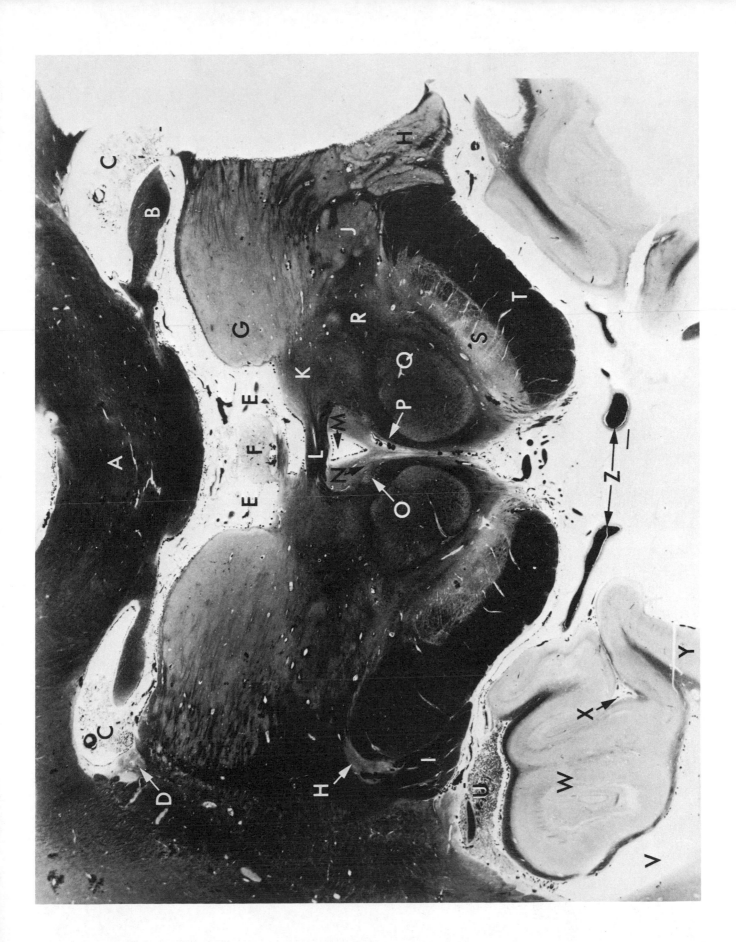

Selected References

TEXTBOOKS

Gilman, S., and S.W. Newman. *Manter and Gatz's Essentials of Clinical Neuroanatomy and Neurophysiology*, 7th ed. F.A. Davis, Philadelphia, 1987.
A very nice, concise overview of the anatomy and physiology of the nervous system — some clinical correlations, too. Recommended strongly as an introductory source of information on the nervous system.

Sidman, R.L., and M. Sidman. *Neuroanatomy: A Programmed Text*. Little, Brown, Boston, 1965.
This is a well-written programmed text and a very painless way to get into the nervous system. I recommend this book very strongly before a neuroanatomy course (either just before or just after reading Gilman and Newman) or before you delve into the central nervous system in detail.

Gardner, E. *Fundamentals of Neurology*, 6th ed. W.B. Saunders, Philadelphia, 1975.
A well-written, integrated, multidisciplinary approach to the foundation of clinical neuroscience. This book serves as an excellent introduction to the structure and function of the nervous system and contains interesting short biographical sketches of important figures in the history of neurology.

deGroot, J., and J.G. Chusid. *Correlative Neuroanatomy*, 20th ed. Appleton and Lange, East Norwalk, CT, 1988.
An intermediate-level, clinically oriented book on neuroanatomy. Useful for quickly reviewing material due to the use of many illustrations and tables.

FitzGerald, M.J.T. *Neuroanatomy: Basic and Applied*. Baillière Tindall, Philadelphia, 1985.
An intermediate-level, clinically and functionally oriented neuroanatomy text. The book includes current concepts concerning nervous system functioning, contains many simple and clear illustrations, and each chapter ends with a section on applied clinical anatomy.

Barr, M.L., and J.A. Kiernan. *The Human Nervous System: An Anatomical Viewpoint*, 5th ed. J.P. Lippincott, Philadelphia, 1988.
An intermediate-level neuroanatomy text suitable for medical students. A very sound text with a helpful appendix on historical figures in neuroscience and a glossary of neuroanatomical terms.

Carpenter, M.B., and J. Sutin. *Human Neuroanatomy*, 8th ed. Williams & Wilkins, Baltimore, 1983.
A more comprehensive textbook for advanced students and for use as a reference source. Recommended for those who are deeply interested in neuroanatomy.

Brodal, A. *Neurological Anatomy in Relation to Clinical Medicine*, 3rd ed. Oxford University Press, New York, 1981.
An authoritative textbook by a highly respected neuroanatomist. This text is useful for the advanced student as well as the neuroscientist seeking a comprehensive presentation of a specific topic. Many references are included.

REVIEW ARTICLES AND MONOGRAPHS

Alexander, G.E., M.R. DeLong, and P.L. Strick. Parallel organization of functionally segregated circuits linking basal ganglia and cortex. *Annu Rev Neurosci* 9:357–381, 1986.

Amaral, D.G., and M.P. Witter. The three-dimensional organization of the hippocampal formation: A review of anatomical data. *Neuroscience* 31:571–591, 1989.

Davidoff, R.A. The dorsal columns. *Neurology* 39:1377–1385, 1989.

Davidoff, R.A. The pyramidal tract. *Neurology* 40:332–339, 1990.

Duvernoy, H.M. *The Human Hippocampus: An Atlas of Applied Anatomy*. Springer-Verlag, New York, 1988.

Englander, R.N., M.G. Netsky, and L.S. Adelman. Location of human pyramidal tract in the internal capsule: Anatomic evidence. *Neurology* 25:823–826, 1975.

Gay, A.J., N.M. Newman, J.L. Keltner, and M.H. Stroud, *Eye Movement Disorders*. C.V. Mosby, St. Louis, 1974.

Gilman, S., J.R. Bloedel, and R. Lechtenberg. *Disorders of the Cerebellum*. F.A. Davis, Philadelphia, 1981.

Haber, S.N. Neurotransmitters in the human and nonhuman primate basal ganglia. *Hum Neurobiol* 5:159–168, 1986.

Humphrey, D.R. Corticospinal systems and their control by premotor cortex, basal ganglia, and cerebellum. Chapter 19 in *Neurobiology*, assoc. ed. W.D. Willis. In *The Clinical Neurosciences*, ed. R.N. Rosenberg. Churchill Livingstone, New York, 1983.

International Anatomical Nomenclature Committee. *Nomina Anatomica*, 6th ed. Churchill Livingstone, New York, 1989.

Jenny, A.B., and C.B. Saper. Organization of the facial nucleus and corticofacial projection in the monkey: A reconsideration of the upper motor neuron facial palsy. *Neurology* 37:930–939, 1987.

Lang, W., J.A. Büttner-Ennever, and U. Büttner. Vestibular projections to the monkey thalamus: An autoradiographic study. *Brain Res* 177:3–17, 1979.

Leichnetz, G.R. The prefrontal cortico-oculomotor trajectories in the monkey: A possible explanation for the effects of stimulation/lesion experiments on eye movement. *J Neurol Sci* 49:387–396, 1981.

Leigh, R.J., and D.S. Zee. *The Neurology of Eye Movements.* F.A. Davis, Philadelphia, 1983.

McGeer, P.L., and E.G. McGeer. Integration of motor func-tions in the basal ganglia in *The Basal Ganglia II: Structure and Function — Current Concepts,* eds. M.B. Carpenter and A. Jayoraman. Plenum Press, New York, 1987.

Nathan, P.W., M.C. Smith, and A.W. Cook. Sensory effects in man of lesions of the posterior columns and of some other afferent pathways. *Brain* 109:1003–1041, 1986.

Index

Supplementary motor area, **66**, **67**, **68**
Synapses, 3

Taste, pathways for, **27**, 27 – 28
Temperature, pathways for, 19 – 21, **20**, 23 – 25, **24**
Temporal lobe, **95**
  coronal sections through, **168 – 169**
  medial, **162 – 163**
  vestibular pathways of, 38, **39**
Tentorium cerebelli, 84, **85**
Thalamostriate vein, **88 – 89**, 90, **137**
Thalamus
  angled horizontal section through, **134 – 135**
  geniculate bodies of. *See* Geniculate bodies of thalamus
  nuclei of. *See* Nuclei, of thalamus
  pulvinar of, **113**, **135**, **167**, **173**, **222**, **223**
Touch, pathways for
  discriminative (fine), 21 – 23, **22**, 25, **26**
  light (crude), 19 – 21, **20**, 23 – 25, **24**
Tracts
  central tegmental, **27**, 28, **62**, **212 – 221**
  corticopontine, 61
  cuneocerebellar, 57, **58**
  dentatorubrothalamic, 61, **129**, **220**, **221**
  dorsolateral, 19, **189**, **194**, **195**
  frontopontine, **216**, **217**, **220**, **221**
  geniculocalcarine, 31, **32**, **33**
  habenulopeduncular, **220**, **221**
  mamillothalamic, **131**, **157**
  olfactory, 28, **29**, **105**, **107**, **151**
  optic, 31, **32**, **33**, **35**, **101**, **107**, **111**, **126**, **129**, **131**,
    154, **157**, **159**, **173**, **222**, **223**
  pyramidal, 46 – 52, **167**, **179**, **181**, **202 – 207**
    corticonuclear (corticobulbar), **45**, 46 – 49, **47**, **216**, **217**,
      220, **221**
    corticospinal, **9**, **45**, 46, 50 – 52, **51**, **52**, **189 – 193**,
      198, **199**, **216**, **217**, **220**, **221**
    decussation of, **198 – 199**
  reticulospinal, 15, 55, **56**
    medullary, 46, **56**, **192**, **193**
    pontine, 46, **56**, **192**, **193**
  rubrospinal, **9**, 46, 59, **60**
  solitary, **27**, 28, **200 – 207**
  spinocerebellar
    anterior, **9**, 57, **58**, **189 – 193**, **198 – 205**
    posterior, **9**, 15, 23, 57, **58**, **192**, **193**, **198 – 203**
  spinocervical, 23
  spinothalamic, **9**, 13, 15, 19, **192**, **193**
  temporoparieto – occipitopontine, **216**, **217**, **220**, **221**
  of trigeminal nerve
    dorsal, 26
    mesencephalic, 25, **212 – 215**
    spinal, 23, **24**, **198 – 211**
  trigeminothalamic, **24**, 25, **26**, **212**, **213**
  vestibulospinal, **9**, 15, 38, **39**, **46**, **54**, 55

Trapezoid body, 36, **37**, **210 – 213**
Trigeminal nerve (V), 5, 6, 7, 15, 49, 84, **99**, **105**, **111**,
    176, **212 – 213**
  See also Nuclei, of trigeminal nerve; Tracts, of trigeminal
    nerve
Trochlear nerve (IV), 5, 6, 7, 44, 84, **105**, **111**, **113**
Tuber cinereum, **111**, **121**, **173**

Uncus, 28, **29**, **107**, **109**, **155**, **173**, **175**
Utricle, 38, **39**

Vagus nerve (X), 6, 7, 8, **27**, 28, **47**, 49, **99**, **111**, **113**
Venous lacunae, 84
Venous return
  from brain, 84 – 90
  from spinal cord, 91, **92**
Venous sinuses of dura mater, 84 – 89
  cavernous, 84, **85**
  confluens of, 84, **85**, **86 – 89**
  intercavernous (circular), 84, **85**
  occipital, 84
  petrosal
    inferior, 84
    superior, 84, **85**, **86 – 89**
  sagittal
    inferior, 84, **85**
    superior, 84, **85**, **144**
  sigmoid, 84, **85**
  sphenoparietal, 84, **85**
  straight, 84, **85**, **86 – 89**, **136**
  transverse, 84, **85**, **86 – 89**
Ventricle, lateral
  collateral trigones of, **138 – 139**, **166 – 167**
  inferior horn of, **166 – 167**, **174**, **175**
  posterior horn of, **138**, **168 – 169**
Vermis, **59**, **177**
Vertebral artery, **72**, 74 – 75, **80 – 83**, **99**
Vestibular (archicerebellar) connections, 52 – 55, **53 – 56**
Vestibular nerve, **39**, **53**, **54**, **59**
Vestibular pathways, 38, **39**
Vestibulocochlear nerve (VIII), 5, 6, 7, 36, 38, **103**, **105**,
    111, **113**, **206 – 209**
Vibration, pathways for, 21 – 23, **22**
Vision, pathways for, 31, **32**, **33**
Visual association areas, 31
Visual cortex, 31, **32**, **33**
Visual reflexes, 7, 34, **35**
Voluntary eye movements. *See* Saccadic eye movements

White matter, 3
White ramus communicans, **9**